## Praise for *Bey(...)*

"*Beyond Sugar Shock* gives you everything yc(...) (...) health into your life . . . without the risk of sugar!" – (...) r of the *New York Times* bestsellers *Women's Bodies, W(...)* (...) *Menopause*

"Sugar is not good for your brain. It increases erratic brain cell firing, pro(...) inflammation, and is clearly addictive. *Beyond Sugar Shock* can help you get sugar out of your life and replace it with health and vitality. It is a powerful program full of easy tips and tactics." — **Daniel G. Amen, M.D.**, best-selling author of *Change Your Brain, Change Your Life*

"*Beyond Sugar Shock* fearlessly tackles the nation's number-one health crisis: the diabesity epidemic. Connie Bennett offers real-life solutions, recipes, take-action programs, and spot-on science to help break the sugar addiction that is fueling our nation's health epidemic." — **Ann Louise Gittleman, Ph.D., C.N.S.**, author of *The Fat Flush Plan and Fat Flush for Life*

"This enjoyable book shows you how to change your diet, reduce your sugar intake, lose weight, and enjoy greater energy than ever before." — **Brian Tracy**, author of *Earn What You're Really Worth*

"If you are ready to love yourself and your body, abandon the wounds of your past, and free yourself from unhealthy addictions, then read *Beyond Sugar Shock*." — **Bernie Siegel, M.D.**, author of *A Book of Miracles* and *Faith, Hope, and Healing*

"Connie Bennett's *Beyond Sugar Shock* is a valuable and important addition to the growing literature on sugar addiction." — **Jonny Bowden, Ph.D., CNS**, author of *Living Low Carb* and *The 150 Healthiest Foods on Earth*

"This refreshing and enlightening book shows how to release sugar addiction easily. It can save your life. Read it!" — **Dr. Joe Vitale**, author of *The Attractor Factor*

"Get this book or risk being trapped in a sugar roller coaster for years to come—or getting diabetes, cancer, and other deadly diseases." — **Mark Sisson**, founder of Mark's Daily Apple and author of *The Primal Blueprint 21-Day Total Body Transformation*

"Tired of being a sugar junkie? Ready to feel better instead of guilty? Then this book is for you. Connie Bennett, Sugar Freedom Coach extraordinaire, will show you how to ditch your sugar addiction by treating your body, mind, and spirit with tenderness, compassion, and even humor!" — **Jacob Teitelbaum, M.D.**, integrative physician and author of *Beat Sugar Addiction Now!*

"As I've discovered myself, one of the keys to being happy is eating well, which includes limiting sugar consumption. But as any sugar addict knows, this is a tough habit to kick! In *Beyond Sugar Shock*, Connie Bennett shows you an easy and empowering way to say farewell to those 'sweet poisons.'" — **Marci Shimoff**, *New York Times* best-selling author of *Happy for No Reason* and *Love for No Reason*

"If you're a sugar addict like most people, you need to read *Beyond Sugar Shock*. This compassionate, comforting, uplifting book will change your life." — **Kathy Smith**, International Fitness Expert

CALGARY PUBLIC LIBRARY

NOV - 2012

*"Beyond Sugar Shock* ambitiously breaks new ground in the field of sugar addiction! Connie shows you how to bravely and easily shift away from negative and harmful thinking to positive and productive thinking to help get you healthier and happier. You must read this book if you are serious about making a change in your health and lifestyle to finally live the life you want and, more importantly, deserve!" — **John Assaraf,** *New York Times* best-selling author of *The Answer and Having It All* and star of the blockbuster movie *The Secret*

"This book will take you on a fun, exciting, transformative six-week adventure, from which you'll emerge healthier, sexier, slimmer, and happier. Plus, you'll finally feel free!" — **Colette Baron-Reid,** internationally renowned intuitive coach and author of *The Map*

"If you have a sugar addiction, who should you turn to for help? Someone who walks their talk and has been there, too! In her book, *Beyond Sugar Shock*, Connie Bennett—a journalist and former sugar-addict-turned-life-and-health-coach—presents a brilliant, foolproof plan to rescue you even if you've been trapped for years." — **Janet Bray Attwood,** co-author of the *New York Times* bestseller *The Passion Test*

"Finally, a book that teaches you to let go of sugar addiction by following a personal body, mind, and spirit program that gets to the emotional core of sugar addiction." — **Brigitte Mars,** author of *Rawsome!*

*"Beyond Sugar Shock* is full of soul-satisfying tools you can implement immediately to nourish your natural, innate desire for a sweeter life. A must-read!" — **Donna Gates,** author of *The Body Ecology Diet* and *The Baby Boomer Diet*

*"Beyond Sugar Shock* gives you a new way to improve your health, love your food, and enjoy your life without the pain." — **Alex Jamieson,** certified health coach, healthy gourmet chef, and author of *The Great American Detox Diet* and *Vegan Cooking for Dummies*

*"Beyond Sugar Shock* is fabulous! It's loaded with secrets to for you to release your sugar addiction. Follow this program and break free to real happiness and joy!" — **Diana Kirschner, Ph.D.,** author of *Love in 90 Days* and *Sealing the Deal*

"If we as a nation are going to stop the obesity crisis, we must overcome our addiction to sugar. We have raised a generation of children, who think sugary cereals, chocolate milk, gummy candies, and the like are part of every meal. *Beyond Sugar Shock*—with its powerful tips, stories, and recipes—is an important tool in the fight against obesity." — **Ann Cooper,** "The Renegade Lunch Lady" and author of *Lunch Lessons*

"Connie's book *Beyond Sugar Shock* is exactly what people need. Get this book and save your waistline, your relationships, your moods, and even your life." — **Brian Alman, Ph.D.,** best-selling weight-loss expert and author of *The Voice*

"An engaging, interactive approach to losing weight in which the reader not only becomes an active participant but becomes the conductor to gain control of his or her own health. Bravo, Connie!" — **Richard J. Johnson, M.D.,** Tomas Berl Professor of Medicine, Chief, Division of Renal Diseases and Hypertension, University of Colorado, Denver, and author of *The Sugar Fix*

"To everyone who has a sugar problem—and that's almost all of us—you must read this remarkable book!" — **Roberta Ruggiero**, President/Founder of The Hypoglycemia Support Foundation, Inc., and author of *The Do's and Don'ts of Hypoglycemia*

"Experts have shown that every effective health change always has better success with a concrete plan, and this book does just that." — **Roberta Lee, M.D.**, Vice Chair, Department of Integrative Medicine, Continuum Center for Health and Healing, Beth Israel Medical Center, and author of *The SuperStress Solution*

"Quitting sugar is no easy feat, but Connie Bennett's life-changing book, *Beyond Sugar Shock*, makes it simple, fun, and do-able. I'll be recommending this book to my clients." — **JJ Virgin, Ph.D.**, Celebrity Fitness Nutrition and Fitness Expert, author of *Six Weeks to Sleeveless and Sexy*, and co-star of the TLC reality series "Freaky Eaters"

"Are you hooked on sugar and fed up with your excess weight? *Beyond Sugar Shock* is the only book you'll ever need on the subject. Read it, and you'll release your addiction at long last—and be able to get a balanced, peaceful, delicious life in the process." — **Lauren Mackler**, author of the bestseller *Solemate*

"Connie Bennett's Sugar Shock! is one of the best books ever written about the toll taken by excess sugar consumption, and *Beyond Sugar Shock* is a worthy and logical follow-up. I give it my highest recommendation."— **Jeff O'Connell,** Bodybuilding.com Editor-in-Chief, author of *Sugar Nation*

"Thank you, Connie, for writing *Beyond Sugar Shock*. I love how easy to read yet informative it is!" — **Patricia Moreno,** Founder, intenSati, and author of *The intenSati Method*

"*Beyond Sugar Shock* answers a huge hunger millions have for an easy way out of their horrible sugar addiction. You're changing people's lives with your powerful, amazing books." — **Kathie Dolgin** (a.k.a. "High Voltage"), health and wellness pioneer and founder of the first sugar-free public school in New York

"With an approach filled with the right ingredients—good facts, smart suggestions, and topped with a little Vitamin L, Love, *Beyond Sugar Shock* is a powerful tool for transforming your health, weight, and happiness." — **Marc David**, best-selling author of *Nourishing Wisdom* and *The Slow Down Diet* and Founder of the Institute for the Psychology of Eating

"*Beyond Sugar Shock* masterfully shows us how to finally get control our sugar or carb addictions—and go from self-loathing to self-love." — **Ken Druck, Ph.D.**, pioneer of life coaching and author of *The Real Rules of Life*

"For many years, Connie Bennett has been warning us of the dangers of what she describes as 'Sugar Shock!' Now she takes you 'beyond' your sweet obsession on a journey to healthy healing using her effective six-week plan that engages your Mind, Body, and Spirit." — **Jimmy Moore,** founder of Livin' La Vida Low-Carb blog and author of *21 Life Lessons From Livin' La Vida Low-Carb*

"As a physician for more than two decades, I've seen firsthand the many diseases sugar addiction can cause and the incredible difficulties patients face in overcoming it—although they know it can be deadly. All sugar addicts need to read *Beyond Sugar Shock*. I'm recommending it to all my patients." — **Keith R. DeOrio, M.D.**, integrative physician

"Connie Bennett has done it again! I strongly recommend this book for anyone seeking solutions for how to make at least 100 years of quality life through good nutrition!" — **Russ Bianchi**, Managing Director and CEO, Adept Solutions, Inc.

"Wow! *Beyond Sugar Shock* is a must-read book for millions of overweight and sugar-addicted people worldwide. At the end of this six-week program, you'll wonder why you ever wanted sweets in the first place, because your life will be so much happier, fuller, and healthier without those nasty insulin-blasting nonfoods." — **Oz Garcia, Ph.D.**, Celebrity Nutrition Expert, whose clients include Oscar winner Hilary Swank and singer Roberta Flack

"People crave sweetness in their lives, but as Connie Bennett wisely points out, you have many more choices than refined sugar. If you've substituted sugar for love, you can find out how to get the real thing by following Connie's six-week plan." — **Carolyn Dean M.D., N.D.**, creator of the Completement Now! Online Wellness Program

"A respected pioneer in this field, Connie packages her considerable experience and knowledge with her always spunky writing style in a motivating, readable, invaluable book." — **Jill Escher**, author of *Farewell, Club Perma-Chub* and founder of www.EndSugarAddiction.com

"*Beyond Sugar Shock* is a must-read for everyone who's got a sweet tooth that just won't quit. Connie will show you how to say *no* with sass, so you can say *yes* to more life." — **Stacey Morgenstern and Carey Peters**, Creators of Holistic MBA

"Kicking your sugar addiction is one of the most difficult challenges on the path to healthier eating. *Beyond Sugar Shock* provides you with a powerful and valuable program to do it once and for all." — **Jared Koch**, nutritional consultant and founder of *Clean Plates* guides

"As a health expert and hypnotherapist, I know how tough it is for people to quit sugar and processed carbs. But Connie Bennett has made the process smooth, simple, and powerful in her book *Beyond Sugar Shock*. You must read this book if you're among millions who can't say no to cookies or candies." — **Mark Patrick**, author of *Wake Up Skinny*

"Connie really walks her talk—and has since 1998! *Beyond Sugar Shock* will help you easily kick your sugar habit to the curb so you can become healthy and whole both inside and out." — **Cynthia Rowland**, facial fitness expert

"*Beyond Sugar Shock* gives us the tools and techniques to deal with our sugar addiction and affliction. Connie empowers us to move beyond our need for sugar, and in the process, she helps us create a life of balance and health." — **Jill R. Baron, M.D.**, integrative physician and functional medicine specialist

# Beyond
## SUGAR
## SHOCK

## ALSO BY CONNIE BENNETT

*Sugar Shock! How Sweets and Simple Carbs Can Derail Your Life—and How You Can Get Back on Track,* with Stephen T. Sinatra, M.D.

# Beyond
## SUGAR
## SHOCK

THE **6-WEEK PLAN** TO BREAK FREE OF
YOUR SUGAR ADDICTION & GET
**SLIMMER, SEXIER, & SWEETER**

# CONNIE BENNETT, CHHC, CPC, ACC

Foreword by Joshua Rosenthal, MScEd, Founder
and Director, Institute for Integrative Nutrition

Recipes & Meal Planning by Jill Lane, C.N.C.

HAY HOUSE

Carlsbad, California • New York City
London • Sydney • Johannesburg
Vancouver • Hong Kong • New Delhi

Copyright © 2012 by Connie Bennett

*Published and distributed in the United States by:* Hay House, Inc.: www.hayhouse.com • *Published and distributed in Australia by:* Hay House Australia Pty. Ltd.: www.hayhouse.com.au • *Published and distributed in the United Kingdom by:* Hay House UK, Ltd.: www.hayhouse.co.uk • *Published and distributed in the Republic of South Africa by:* Hay House SA (Pty), Ltd.: www.hayhouse.co.za • *Distributed in Canada by:* Raincoast: www.raincoast.com • *Published in India by:* Hay House Publishers India: www.hayhouse.co.in

*Design:* Tricia Breidenthal

All rights reserved. No part of this book may be reproduced by any mechanical, photographic, or electronic process, or in the form of a phonographic recording; nor may it be stored in a retrieval system, transmitted, or otherwise be copied for public or private use—other than for "fair use" as brief quotations embodied in articles and reviews—without prior written permission of the publisher.

The author of this book does not dispense medical advice or prescribe the use of any technique as a form of treatment for physical, emotional, or medical problems without the advice of a physician, either directly or indirectly. The intent of the author is only to offer information of a general nature to help you in your quest for emotional and spiritual well-being. In the event you use any of the information in this book for yourself, which is your constitutional right, the author and the publisher assume no responsibility for your actions.

Precautions have been taken to protect and disguise any confidential, personally identifiable information concerning persons discussed in this book.

### Library of Congress Cataloging-in-Publication Data

Bennett, Connie.
  Beyond sugar shock : the 6-week plan to break free of your sugar addiction & get slimmer, sexier, & sweeter / Connie Bennett ; foreword by Joshua Rosenthal ; recipes & meal planning by Jill Lane.
    p. cm.
  Includes bibliographical references and index.
  ISBN 978-1-4019-3189-6 (pbk. : alk. paper) 1. Sugar--Pathophysiology. 2. Carbohydrates, Refined--Pathophysiology. 3. Nutritionally induced diseases. 4. Food habits. 5. Physical fitness--Nutritional aspects. I. Lane, Jill. II. Title.
  RC627.R43B44 2012
  616.3'998--dc23
                        2012001566

**Tradepaper ISBN:** 978-1-4019-3189-6
**Digital ISBN:** 978-1-4019-3190-2

15  14  13  12   4  3  2  1
1st edition, June 2012

Printed in the United States of America

SUSTAINABLE FORESTRY INITIATIVE
Certified Chain of Custody
Promoting Sustainable Forestry
www.sfiprogram.org
SFI-01268

SFI label applies to the text stock

### To My Beloved Mom

*To my amazingly strong, talented, inspiring mom. Thank you for teaching me by your stellar example to believe in myself and to optimistically pursue my goals and dreams, to embrace the arts and other passions with a childlike enthusiasm, and to persevere no matter what.*

### To My Medical Saviors, Because of Whom I'm Here to Help You

*To Roberta Ruggiero and Keith DeOrio, M.D., who "saved my life" in April 1998 by encouraging me to quit my dangerous addiction to sugar and quickie carbs.*

### To Millions of You Sugar and Carb Addicts Around the World

*To millions of discouraged, desperate, distressed sugar and carb addicts of all ages and sizes—who hate "needing" tempting desserts or processed carbohydrates.*

*To my many bold, committed coaching clients and members of my Sugar Freedom Now Course (or Break Free of Your Sugar Addiction in 6 Weeks Program) over the years. I couldn't have written this book without your brilliant ideas, insights, and questions.*

*To all sugar sufferers and carb cravers, my deepest desire is that* Beyond Sugar Shock *gives you the simple, doable plan you crave so you can easily, effortlessly dissolve your harmful sugar or carb habit for good and become your authentic, slim, sexy, happy, healthy self, and get the sweeterlicious (my word for sweeter, luscious, scrumptious, and delicious) life that you so richly deserve.*

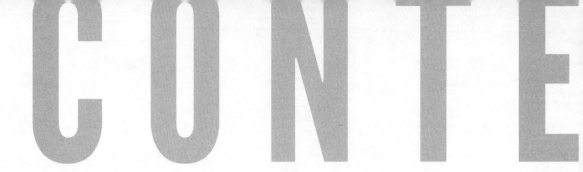

NTS

# FOREWORD

Imagine a caveman walking through today's supermarket looking for something to eat. As he hunts up and down the aisles, he gets more and more frustrated by all the boxes, cans, and jars because he has absolutely no clue what to do with them. Unless he comes across the meat counter or produce section, the poor guy will starve.

It's a wasteland out there. You've got to fight your way past all the nutrient-stripped, overly processed fake foods—the breads, crackers, chips, candies, and cakes, as well as the frozen-this and stovetop-that, which all compose the Standard American Diet (S.A.D.). American consumers have developed a taste for processed foods that are far removed from their origins. Our ancestors would barely recognize the food in our shopping carts.

The truth is that many people have become disconnected from real, whole foods, and they have lost touch with the reality that our food comes from the earth, or from live animals that roam the land or fish that swim in the sea. Rarely do people think about the fact that what they eat profoundly affects how they think, how they act, and how they perform in their daily lives.

Pause for a moment and think about how you feel at different times of the day. For instance, do you tend to feel exhausted or scattered soon after lunch? Come late afternoon, do you crash and crave candies, cookies, or soda? Or do you get cranky or irritable between meals?

Let's face it. It's *the norm* these days to be a sugar or carb addict. Look around you: who doesn't have a tortured love affair with processed sugar and refined carbohydrates? It's become very easy to reach for the most accessible sweet treat, but it's also become increasingly difficult to understand and manage these cravings. So how do you break free from the vicious sugar cycle?

You've just taken the first step. The book you're now holding in your hands can help you transform your relationship with those chemicalized sweets and processed carbs and find a much happier, healthier life in the process.

Beyond Sugar Shock will not only help you to rise above your sugar addiction, but it will also show you how to do so gently, gracefully, and compassionately. Connie has created a comprehensive approach that helps you activate what she calls *The Sweetness Principle,* which helps you make peace with your cravings and have fun in the process. She also gives you brilliant, innovative tools to fill yourself up in deeper, more profound ways so you can find long-lasting, more satisfying, true nourishment.

In 2005, I had the pleasure of watching Connie study and grow as a student at the Institute for Integrative Nutrition. While at IIN, Connie demonstrated a deep-seated passion for helping people let go of their sugar addiction so they could lead better lives and make a difference.

In recent years, I've proudly watched her become an internationally recognized "Sugar Freedom Coach," best-selling author of *Sugar Shock!* (her first book), and one of the world's leading sugar addiction experts. She's a sought-after motivating speaker and a powerful life and health coach, too.

Throughout this book, Connie will guide you step by step to create a balanced life. You will learn how to nurture your body, create a happy mind that's full of joyous and optimistic thoughts, and elevate your spirit. Are you ready to begin?

Let me congratulate you, because you're now on track to create a life that's sweeter, delicious, luscious, and more sensuous—what Connie calls *sweeterlicious.*

That's *really* the American dream, isn't it?

**Joshua Rosenthal**
**Founder and Director**
**Institute for Integrative Nutrition**

# A WARM WELCOME FROM YOUR ONCE SUGAR-ADDICTED AUTHOR

## YOUR AMAZING LIFE AWAITS!

*"If you've been addicted to a harmful substance, to overeating, or even to being a doormat, listen to the voice within that begs you to be big rather than small, and take one corrective step."*

— DR. WAYNE W. DYER, PH.D., AUTHOR OF *THE POWER OF INTENTION*

Greetings, wonderful readers. Welcome. I invite you to imagine that I'm giving you a warm, joyful, congratulatory hug because you're about to embark on what could be the most exciting adventure of your life.

Today's a really big day for you. You've taken a huge step by picking up this book. Be proud of yourself for stepping out of your comfort zone by making the smart, conscious choice to speed Beyond Sugar Shock and *Get a Sweeter Life Naturally,* as I put it.

As we begin our transformational journey together, I urge you to trust the inner intelligence that guided you to me and this six-week program.

Without a doubt, you're here for a very important reason. Whether you or someone close to you got this book for you, the fact that you're reading it now means that no matter how long or how much you've been struggling with your addiction to sugar or processed carbs, you're finally ready to triumph over them both for good.

And you will! I have complete confidence in you. I fully believe that by the time you finish this program, your sugar and carb habit will begin to feel like a sad, distant memory and a valuable lesson. And if you have weight issues, you'll be well on your way to having *less* of you—which means that you'll have *more* of a life.

Together we'll go on a thrilling, fulfilling, interactive escapade that engages, motivates, and nurtures you. This six-week program will help you appreciate, honor, respect, and approve of your body; revitalize, refresh, and renew yourself; improve your concentration and become more productive; boost your metabolism and moods; peel off those extra unwanted pounds that may have been plaguing you for years; rev up your libido (yes, this can happen!); recharge your relationships; put your health back on track; and heighten your pleasure in just about everything you choose to do.

In this book, we'll celebrate wholesome, quality foods, because when you let go of your junk-food habit, you'll begin to relish clean, healthy foods. You'll also be getting a compassionate, far-reaching, life-changing Mind-Body-Spirit program, which offers you easy tools and tactics to bring all of your thoughts, emotions, spirituality, and physical needs into alignment.

That's what makes *Beyond Sugar Shock* so different. Most books about how to change what you eat and lose weight focus almost exclusively on what you put in your mouth and how much you exercise. After spending well over a decade educating, inspiring, and coaching sugar and carb addicts like you and creating tips and techniques to keep you gleefully sugar-free, I've discovered that adjusting what you eat or how much you move isn't nearly enough to help you totally release your carb addiction.

Trust me, your Mind matters, too. You're far more likely to complete this program successfully and make permanent changes to the way you eat if you maintain a positive attitude and mind-set over the next six weeks. That means staying happy, engaged, and focused as you move from one week's activities to the next.

Later, I'll also show you some fantastic ways to control those insidious mind games otherwise known as *cravings*. Now that you're kicking sugar, cravings may hit, so you want to be prepared.

Okay, so Body and Mind probably make a lot of sense to you. But Spirit? After all, you just want to quit sugar or shed weight, not become a woo-woo, airy-fairy person, right? Let me explain.

Most sugar addicts, I've noticed, are steeped, mired, and entrapped in negative thought patterns. For one thing, they're often overly focused on their bodies or weight. Their self-disgust is almost palpable. In fact, when people first come to me for help, they often say things like, "*I hate my body*" or "*I detest my big belly.*" They also believe that quitting their heavily entrenched habit is close to impossible. They'll say, "*I just can't envision life without my favorite sugary snacks.*"

That's why just addressing your Mind and Body isn't nearly enough. To truly make *lasting peace* with your sugar or carb relationship—and to rise above it and let it go—you also need to address your Spirit. By that word, I mean two things. First, your goal is to regularly fill up on activities that nourish and replenish you. For instance, you'll need to get both sufficient Vitamin Z (sleep) and physical activity. Both will lift your Spirit.

Once you've boosted your morale, you've set the stage to take yourself to an even higher plane so you can *really* focus on your Spirit. Doing such enriching activities as meditation, forgiveness, gratitude, or yoga will soothe you, lift your moods, and strengthen your ability to happily and gracefully follow through with this program. You may even begin to experience more joy and freedom, feel more connected to your higher consciousness, and become more eager to pursue your passions.

Letting go of your addictions will allow you to get a yummy, sweeter, delicious, scrumptious, luscious, sensuous life—one that I call *sweeterlicious*. You'll also experience an exhilarating feeling of liberation from your sugar addiction, as many of my private and group coaching clients, as well as thousands of Sugar Kickers I've helped worldwide, have discovered.

## Are You the Right Reader?

Now, let me help you find out if you're in the right place. Depending on your particular situation, you may fall into one or more categories. You're the right reader if:

- You're among the millions of adult Americans—two-thirds of the population—who are struggling with weight issues and who want to shed their unwanted pounds for good, to both look and feel better.

- You feel downright *addicted* to sugary foods or processed, white-flour carbs, much like an alcoholic or drug addict. (You may even refer to yourself as a *carbaholic, chocoholic, sugar addict,* or *sugaraholic.*)

- You think a good breakfast consists of a Danish roll or a bowl of sweet cereal, orange juice, and a cup of sugar-filled coffee.

- You're rarely or never in the mood for sex.

- You're a woman of any age, who has a variety of female challenges. For instance, you feel like *&+^% before and during your period. Or perhaps you've been unable to conceive. Or, if you're going through menopause, you may experience intense symptoms such as hot flashes, memory lapses, and night sweats.

- You're suffering from fibromyalgia, chronic fatigue, or persistent yeast infections.

- You or someone you love has one of what I call *The Preventable Big Killers*—heart disease, type 2 diabetes, or Alzheimer's disease—and you don't want to die before your time.

- You've read my book *Sugar Shock!* and although it convinced you to quit your dangerous habit, you'd still like more guidance.

- You're suffering from one or more of the many perplexing symptoms of hypoglycemia or low blood sugar, such as mood swings, crying spells, severe fatigue, headaches, forgetfulness, restlessness, light-headedness, nightmares, mental confusion, anxiety, depression, heart palpitations, digestive problems, muscle or joint pains, cold hands and feet, and the chills.

- You want to look and feel younger and get more vitality, stamina, and exuberance.

So welcome, all of you Right Readers.

## Are You Trapped in S.A.D.?

Before our six weeks together are up, you'll look back on your life before stopping sugar as a time when you were S.A.D.: unhappily trapped in the Standard American Diet. For many Americans, this diet consists of prepackaged, nutrient-deprived, fiber-poor, highly processed cereals, breads, cookies, crackers, cakes, candies, and pasta—often loaded with sugar.

Nowadays, for the typical person in the United States, almost one-quarter of his or her diet is S.A.D.—i.e. "junk food." According to one analysis of the habits of 4,760 adults, soft drinks were the #1 source of calories. In fact, sweets and desserts, soft drinks, and alcoholic beverages made up nearly 25 percent of participants' total calorie intake. Next came more S.A.D. foods such as potato chips and other salty snacks and fruit-flavored drinks, which, along with pizza and hamburgers, added another 5 percent of calories.

"We knew people are eating a lot of junk food, but to have one-quarter to *almost one-third* of their calories coming from these categories is appalling," observed lead researcher Gladys Block, Ph.D., a professor of epidemiology and public health nutrition at the University of California at Berkley's School of Public Health.

Meanwhile, S.A.D. also means that you're putting a lot of other dangerous things into your lovely body, including high-fructose corn syrup (a popular sweetener added to thousands of processed products and which research has linked to such health hazards as obesity and metabolic syndrome); hydrogenated oils (unhealthy fats found in many processed foods); phytic acid (which is contained in most grains, beans, nuts, and seeds, and considered an *antinutrient* because it reduces your absorption of valuable vitamins and minerals); acrylamide (a carcinogenic chemical that can form in carbs and starchy foods such as potato chips, French fries, and cereal products when heated above 248 degrees Fahrenheit); sodium nitrate (a preservative used in processed meats that may increase your risk for heart disease and cancer of the colon, breast, prostate, and pancreas); and monosodium glutamate, or MSG (a class of chemicals known as *excitotoxins*, which are added to many processed foods and may lead to various chronic diseases).

When you repeatedly eat these processed, sugary foods or sugar-filled carbs (what I call *quickie carbs, culprit carbs,* and *toxic carbs,* among other phrases) and other S.A.D. nonfoods, you're putting yourself in danger. (Soon, you'll learn some of the ways how.)

## What to Expect in *Beyond Sugar Shock*

Just *eliminating* sweets and quickie carbs (or mostly cutting them out) will radically improve your life. You'll be surprised at how far-reaching the changes will be.

You'll soon begin to automatically choose, and even prefer, pure, fresh, quality foods. You'll know more about where your meals come from, and won't need to squint to decipher the fine print in a long list of ingredients on food labels, because you'll be eating fresh foods or packaged foods with fewer added items.

In addition, you'll join millions of like-minded people worldwide, who are committed to what many call *natural foods:* mostly organic, wholesome foods, as close to their natural state as possible. For instance, while writing this book, I made weekly trips to a farmers' market, where I found yummy dark purple and yellow carrots; delicious maroon beans; crunchy sunflower greens; delicious Kirby cucumbers; and many aromatic herbs such as rosemary, stevia, spearmint, basil, dill, rosemary, and oregano; and lemon balm, which added zest to my meals.

Even if your life now revolves around culprit carbs, and you rarely cook or can't even imagine getting out a salad bowl, much less a garlic press, I predict that you—along with your kids, sweetheart, significant other, and even some friends—will soon enjoy shopping and whipping up lip-smacking, nutritious meals made from real, alive foods.

When you consciously choose to eat and drink in this higher, more evolved way, you'll also find yourself naturally opting for positive, nourishing thoughts, too. This, in turn, will allow you to experience a more enchanting, wholesome life in which you achieve a balance of your Mind, Body, and Spirit.

Within six weeks, you'll be amazed at the fulfilled, empowered, healthier person you've become. I invite you now to let your imagination run free. Picture the profound feeling of fun, joy, and excitement that will be yours in a month and a half.

Imagine how you'll feel when you slip into your skinnier jeans, exuberantly enjoy your favorite activities, embrace self-loving habits, gleefully bound (rather than wearily drag yourself) into hot bedroom action with your sweetheart, and be on the fast track to an intoxicating sugar-free life.

**YOU'RE A HAPPY, SUCCESSFUL SUGAR KICKER WHEN . . .**
You admit that your life is now very S.A.D.—but you're ready for it to be SWEET!

## Terms to Help You Glide from Sugar Shock to Sugar Freedom

Before we move on, let me give you a quick overview of important concepts and common terms I present within the book.

### SUGAR SHOCK!

This is an easily avoidable, health-harming, mood-damaging, confusion-creating constellation of symptoms that afflicts millions worldwide. You probably put yourself into Sugar Shock frequently—possibly several times a day—by repeatedly over-consuming sugar and other processed, nutrient-deprived sweet foods. On average, you overdose on sugar to the tune of some 150 pounds per year, if you go by the low United States Department of Agriculture (USDA) calculations. Bear in mind, though, that your consumption may be far higher. If you consider insider figures, each of you may be mindlessly taking in as many as 228 pounds of sweeteners, including high-fructose corn syrup, crystalline fructose, inulin, corn syrup solids, dextrose, maltodextrin, beet sugar, cane sugar, maltose, and others. In addition to all those sweeteners, you may be unthinkingly consuming nearly 200 pounds per year of sugar's culpable cousins: refined white-flour products, such as white bread, white rice, sweetened cereals, white-flour pasta, and chips—or what I call *much-like-sugar carbs, toxic carbs,* or *quickie carbs,* among other terms. Frequently playing Sugar Shock roulette can trigger chronically elevated blood-sugar levels, repeatedly over-stimulate insulin release, cause excessive inflammation, and pave the way for nearly 150 devastating, mostly preventable conditions or diseases, including obesity, type 2 diabetes, blood-sugar disorders, heart disease, cancer, and even Alzheimer's, among others. If you're in Sugar Shock, you also may suffer from fatigue, headaches, depression, anxiety, and irritability. The bottom line is that Sugar Shock can send you speeding toward obesity, disease, and an early death.

## HFCS Shock, or Fructose Shock

Any time you eat foods from a box, can, jar, or package, or dine out at a fast-food place or food chain, there's a good chance you're consuming high-fructose corn syrup (HFCS), which is added to thousands of refined foods, even ones that aren't sweet. Research from Princeton University shows that high-fructose corn syrup is metabolized differently in our bodies than sucrose and that consuming it on such a massive scale—as most of you do—may be *more damaging* than eating foods and beverages that contain sucrose. HFCS Shock, or Fructose Shock, like Sugar Shock, may make you fat and can lead to what are often called diseases of modern civilization such as heart disease, type 2 diabetes, and cancer.

Meanwhile, white powdered, processed fructose, which you can find in health-food stores, isn't any better and is as difficult to metabolize as high-fructose corn syrup, according to Nancy Appleton, Ph.D., author of *Suicide by Sugar: A Startling Look at Our #1 National Addiction.*

Please note, though, that in discussing fructose, I'm not talking about fiber-filled, nutrient-dense fruits, which may contain naturally occurring fructose, galactose, dextrose, sucrose, maltose, lactose, glucose, levulose, pectin, oligosaccharides, antioxidants, phytonutrients, minerals, and beneficial vitamins, according to food scientist Russ Bianchi, managing director and CEO of Adept Solutions, Inc., a global food and beverage product development firm.

## S.A.D.

This is the Standard American Diet. S.A.D. includes Sugar-Shocking and culprit-carb foods, as well as fatty, fried, fiber-poor, nonalive, nutrient-deprived, heavily processed, unhealthy foodstuffs and sugary beverages, including soda, iced teas, and energy drinks. Consuming such a poor diet sets you up for weight gain, disease, and a lifetime of unhappiness—which is why I often use the acronym S.A.D.

## Sugar Shock Freedom

Sugar Shock Freedom is an amazing place where you break the mesmerizing stranglehold that toxic carbs have over you and achieve a now-elusive feeling of independence, excitement, joy, delight, and exhilaration, which is unlike anything you've ever felt.

## SWEET

Throughout this book, you'll find examples of S.A.D. and SWEET. When you leave behind your S.A.D. life, you'll embrace SWEET instead. The acronym stands for Savor Wholesome, Exciting, Energy-producing foods *and* activities that Turn on your better life of Mind-Body-Spirit balance.

## Since 1998, I've Been Training to Help You Break Free of Your Sugar Addiction

Back in spring of 1998, I was very much like you, I imagine. As you'll soon discover, for years, I was a candy-chomping, chips-craving, cookie-crunching, obsessed sugar and carb addict, who regularly, nervously, unthinkingly shoved junk foods filled with dangerous processed sugars and other sweeteners, chemicals, fats, flours, flavorings, and dyes into my poor body. Can you relate?

Worse still, my habit "imprisoned" me—or so it felt. It shattered and strained my health, moods, relationships, concentration, self-esteem, and happiness. In other words, I was stuck in sugary quicksand, as you may be now.

Thankfully, I conquered my sugar addiction, and for 14 years and running (as of this book's publication), I've made it my mission to help others do the same. I've also received training as a certified health coach, certified life coach, natural foods chef, and vision board coach. Most important, since 2002, I've been helping thousands of people around the world successfully bid sugar farewell.

I'm also author of the best-selling book *Sugar Shock!*, which has been praised by Dr. Mehmet Oz, Dr. Christiane Northrup, and many other experts. In the next chapter, you'll learn more about my story and how I made the transition from sour junk-food junkie to happy health guru.

## YOU'RE A HAPPY, SUCCESSFUL SUGAR KICKER WHEN . . .

Someone offers you a frosted cookie (your former favorite) at a party, and it doesn't interest you. You reply, "Thanks for offering, but I'd rather have celery with your amazing homemade hummus. Would you share the recipe, please?"

## Let's Gather in a Huddle to Prepare for Your Win

Now, I invite you to imagine that you're about to play your favorite sport. Please visualize me as your encouraging, ever-enthusiastic, steadfast Sugar Freedom Coach, who emphatically tells you that—despite many previous, upsetting losses—this time, you and your team can and will overturn your losing streak, and finally get the win for which you have been yearning.

See us all together: millions of sugaraholics from around the world gathered in a huddle. There I am, beaming and calmly reassuring you that you're on your way to a juicier, happier, sweeterlicious life, in which you no longer crave, much less desire, those nutrient-robbed, energy-draining carbs and other S.A.D. foods that bring you excess weight, emotional and physical pain, and life-threatening diseases.

Throughout your journey, as your compassionate, loving, I've-been-there coach, remember that I'm always cheering you on and reminding you that when you release your sugar and carb habit, you'll finally get the wondrous life that you desire and deserve.

## Better-than-Prescription-Strength Affirmations Will Ensure Your Success

As you begin your journey, you want to keep an open mind and heart, as well as a positive, can-do attitude. Therefore, throughout this book, you'll find affirmations (inspired by Louise L. Hay) that I've created to help you consciously choose encouraging thoughts and declarations that will move you from Sugar Bondage to Sugar Freedom.

Starting right now, you'll use words and statements that will help you achieve success in this program. A large part of why I triumphed is because I kept telling myself that I was *already* sugar-free and healthy. Essentially, I filled myself up (like you would put gas in your car) with affirmations like *I, Connie, am happy, healthy, and radiant* or *I, Connie, am slim, sensual, and sugar-free.* Day in and day out, I kept repeating these bold affirmations, until eventually they permeated my consciousness. Sure enough, they became true—and still are—and now I'm here to help you years later.

To get the most benefit from this positive practice, repeat each affirmation aloud at least five times, preferably twice a day. (Ideal times are first thing in the morning and right before bedtime.)

Say your favorite affirmations as you go about your day—doing dishes, washing your hair, or waiting in line at the bank—whenever you need them. You'll be surprised at how many times you can slip in affirmations, even if your schedule is jam-packed. Quick tip: whenever possible, as you repeat your affirmation, stand up, spread your arms wide and high, smile, and proclaim your statements joyously, proudly, and emphatically.

Please note that although I'm giving you recommended affirmations, if some of them don't sound like you, just create your own versions that resonate more personally. Shortly, you'll also find out how it's important to *feel* your success at the same time.

### Affirmation: This book is easily helping me kick sugar for good.

### Your Success Is Entirely Up to You

Ultimately, as with any new hobby, relationship, or job, you get back what you put into it. Therefore, your success with this program depends on how much you're invested in it and what you put into it.

You can release your sugar addiction if you keep an open mind and embrace the empowering ideas and life-changing concepts presented here. Make sure to do all the "inner stretching" suggested. By this, I mean undertake all the Adventurcises (my word for adventurous exercises) and Playcises (playful exercises) throughout the book. Most of your growth will happen *when we're apart*—when you put down this book and put these principles into practice. That's when your change will really happen.

To help you along the way, I've also given you powerful tips and tools in *Coach Connie's SWEET Success Strategy* sidebars.

## Fasten Your Seat Belts as You Quickly Move into Your Sweeterlicious Life

It's time to buckle up. *Beyond Sugar Shock* will give you a fast-moving, roller-coaster ride to a slimmer, sexier body, a happier disposition, and a sweeterlicious life. Get ready to be inspired!

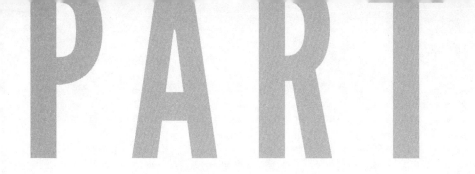

# THE SOUR TRUTH
# ABOUT SWEETS

## CHAPTER 1

# MY S.A.D. TO SWEET STORY

**Affirmation: I'm now rising above my painful sugar past like Connie.**

Never did I imagine in April 1998 that by finally accepting, facing, and releasing my dangerous, disempowering carb addiction, I would become dedicated, determined, and driven to help you, dear readers, release your Sugar Shock.

To be honest with you, I'd much rather bury my dark sugar past for good. I really dislike remembering that terrible time. But I'm sharing my personal story in the hopes that you'll learn from it and be inspired to rise above your sugar misery, too.

As I sit here, still baffled by my former bad-girl sugar behavior, I'm forced to admit that I behaved much like an addict who is hooked on drugs, alcohol, sex, gambling, tobacco, texting, coffee, or another dangerous substance or activity.

In retrospect, it's now evident that while in the grips of my addiction, at times, I may have alienated some of the people closest to me. A few loved ones became so frustrated that they stopped trying to help me, avoided me when possible, or even ended our relationship.

As I piece together and write about these unpleasant memories, I'm still ashamed, shocked, and embarrassed. Thankfully, I have many cool tools (including Ho'oponopono and Tapping) to release any emotional vestiges. (You'll learn them later, too.)

## Sugar Brought on 44 Symptoms and Huge Emotional Torment

During this period in my life in the late 1990s, I was plagued by 44 perplexing physical symptoms. So, on any given day, I'd suffer from ailments like crushing fatigue, persistent migraines, nagging mental confusion, scary heart palpitations, disorienting dizziness, debilitating muscle pains, unpredictable cold hands and feet overpowering sugar cravings, and/or ravenous hunger between meals. Plus, during "that time of the month," I'd endure terrible PMS and menstrual agony. Now that I know better, it's quite obvious: the more sugar I had, the worse my conditions got. Unfortunately, it took years for me to make that connection.

It's also clear now that whenever I was *heavy into the sugar* or *using my drug of choice*—as many sugaraholics describe it even though we're talking about legal foods—I felt imprisoned, incomplete, and miserable.

Disappointment in myself reigned supreme. Depression dogged me. Feelings of angst, anxiety, and melancholy consumed me. Inner peace eluded me. My self-esteem, spirit, and energy levels plummeted whenever I caved in to my cravings, which was often.

And I was one persistent sugar seeker. I would drive across town just to get my favorite hard candies in several flavors. Or I'd go in another direction to buy special gourmet chocolate. And I'd seek out red licorice and tiny crackers at other locations. In short, I was often self-medicating with sugar and quickie carbs. Sound familiar?

But I never got what I *really* wanted, which was sweetness, joy, passion, excitement, confidence, contentment, inner peace, self-pride, and a spiritual connection.

You're probably wondering about how my habit affected my weight since I *used* sugar so often. Unlike what you'd expect, I was not overweight. If you'd met me then, unless you saw me chomping on all that junk, you wouldn't have had a clue that I was addicted to sugar and carbs.

Nonetheless I was horribly malnourished, because I often skimped on quality, nutrient-filled foods and some 40 (or even 50) percent or more of my diet revolved around culprit carbs.

If you're struggling with unwanted weight, let me assure you that just cutting out sugar and processed carbs is *the fast track to weight loss.* And if you're a slim or average-weight sugar addict, as I once was, you may also lose some weight, but most of your many benefits will have to do with how you feel and behave.

## I Make Dreaded Calls to Confront My S.A.D. Past

Given that I was in a spaced-out, sugar-induced fog more than 14 years ago, I had to call people close to me to piece together a clear picture of what I was like back then.

Although I'm an experienced journalist, author, and writer, this was one tough assignment. Who wants to give those you care about carte blanche to unreservedly, brutally dish the truth about the scattered mess you were?

Suffice it to say that during conversations with friends and family members, I repeatedly shook my head in horror, dismay, or remorse; gasped in shock; or laughed uncontrollably. And after getting off the phone to write this, I cried—a lot.

While socked in by double-digit physical ailments and obsessed with candy, I was also experiencing profound, perplexing emotional pain. Friends and family now describe a sad, tormented, moody, out-of-control *Sugar Shrew*.

For instance, my clever, creative friend Darla (not her real name), with whom I spent a lot of time at the height of my sugar addiction, recalls: "I never knew if I was going to get the demon Connie or the angel Connie. You'd start out as very sweet and nice and decent, and I loved hanging out with you, but then, all of a sudden, it's like a switch would go off.

"I was shocked by your mood swings. You'd get really speedy, out of control, brassy, angry, weepy, upset, or uncharacteristically impatient. Then you'd go into an avalanche of uncontrolled, unchecked self-loathing. All this was tough to be around."

Darla also remembers my big candy habit. "You had a huge sugar stash everywhere. One time I opened a drawer, and you jumped at me and yelped, '*Don't touch those. They're mine!*' You were like a dog protecting a favorite bone. In retrospect, I felt that you needed help, but I wasn't sure what kind."

Things got so strained between Darla and me that we stopped talking and eventually lost touch. Years later, around 2002, when I was writing *Sugar Shock!*, I mustered the courage to call her up to apologize and tell her how I'd discovered that my sugar habit was to blame for my peculiar behavior. She then shared that she, too, had sugar issues and knew that her habit may have contributed to her getting breast cancer.

"It's clear now that sugar had you in its clutches. It was your puppeteer," Darla reflected. "But sugar was also your greatest teacher. It allowed you to liberate yourself, make better choices, and find your way back to your genuine inner sweetness."

Thankfully, Darla and I are friends again.

## Tracey Stands by Me Even Though I Become a Sugar Shrew

Now, let's fast-forward to a morning in the spring of 1998, when my good friend Tracey (also a pseudonym) and I had plans to go play in posh Beverly Hills.

But I had a sugar agenda first.

Two hours before meeting Tracey, after skipping breakfast, I swung by my favorite gourmet candy store to buy handfuls of low-calorie hard candies in various flavors (like banana, cinnamon, chocolate, peanut butter, butterscotch, and licorice). And I couldn't pass up on chocolate coconut haystacks and pieces of chocolate-covered honeycomb. In short order, I began devouring them like a defiant kid overdosing on Halloween candies behind her parents' backs.

At first, Tracey and I had fun. We laughed uproariously about our boyfriend challenges while window-shopping on trendy Rodeo Drive. Next, we popped into our favorite department store, where a makeup artist started applying eye shadow and mascara on Tracey. All the while, I was content to polish off more candies.

But suddenly, after about 45 minutes, I became jittery, nervous, dazed, headachy, unfocused, tearful, and panicky. Quickly, I leaned over to them and desperately, quietly pleaded, *"Can you please hurry up and finish? I need to eat now!"*

After the artist hurriedly finished applying Tracey's lipstick, we rushed to a nearby restaurant, where I unthinkingly grumbled at our poor waiter for taking too long.

"You had a major reaction. You snarled at him, became impatient and irritable, and begged for food *now*," Tracey recalls, describing what was undoubtedly a severe hypoglycemic reaction caused by skipping breakfast, glutting myself on sugar, and plummeting blood-sugar levels.

In other words, Tracey witnessed what I call "the sad sugar switch," when the happy, playful, fun Connie vanished and an illogical, emotional, short-fused, high-on-sugar Sugar Shrew took her place, against my will, of course.

Soon, though, after eating a healthy lunch—a piece of whitefish, some dilled pickles, and a vegetable salad, the Sugar Shrew disappeared.

"You completely calmed down and were fun to be around again," Tracey recalls. "You were back to being the reasonable, cheerful Connie I so like."

Despite my occasional Sugar Shrew moments, Tracey stuck by me. "You were still one of my best friends," she says. "But now that you're eating right, I like you so much better."

## My Sugar Education

After the incident with Tracey, my physical problems got so intense I couldn't take it anymore. I found an astute physician, Keith DeOrio, M.D., who knew a lot about nutrition, homeopathy, vitamins, acupuncture, and, as I soon learned, sugar.

To this day, I remember sobbing in his office. Soon, after running some tests, my doctor delivered his diagnosis: reactive hypoglycemia, or low blood sugar.

His solution was straightforward: if I wanted my ailments to go away, I needed to change my diet. Straightforward, sure, but *easy*? No way!

My doctor warned me that if I continued abusing my body with sugar, I could get type 2 diabetes, kidney failure, nerve damage, heart disease, or even cancer.

Although my M.D.'s diagnosis scared me, I just *wasn't ready* to stop eating my favorite sweets and fast carbs. The thought of quitting *The Sweet White Stuff* seemed close to impossible.

*How could I do it?* I wondered. I didn't *want* to give up my beloved chocolate, cinnamon candies, and red licorice! Frankly, the idea of living without my cherished "treats" unsettled and depressed me.

So I didn't follow my doctor's advice right away. But I did take one important step in the right direction: I started reading books about sugar's dangers.

One of the more entertaining memories I have is of me mindlessly gobbling red licorice and hard candies *while reading books* such as *Sugar Blues* by William Dufty, *Lick the Sugar Habit* by Nancy Appleton, Ph.D., and *Get the Sugar Out* by Ann Louise Gittleman, Ph.D., C.N.S.

Remember, it was 1998 and the Internet wasn't as readily accessible as it is today, so I couldn't easily hop online to do research or join a support group late at night when in the throes of a sugar craving.

After a few weeks of learning about sugar's dangers, I suddenly realized that I desperately needed to take action. I had no choice. Unless I quit sugar, I'd be on a fast path to disease and an early death.

Finally, after years of ignoring my inner antisugar guidance system, I started listening, and I began viewing my addiction with the deadly seriousness it deserved.

## I Quit! Life Becomes Sweet: My Ailments Vanish & Connie, the Happy Sugar Kicker, Is Born

Finally, on April 15, 1998, I did the previously unthinkable—at long last, I turned my back on sweets and quickie carbs.

I won't lie to you. It wasn't always easy. Since I quit cold turkey, I had intense withdrawal symptoms. I felt headachy, tired, moody, depressed, and just plain blah. I needed to nap a lot. (Thankfully, as a freelance journalist, I could cut back on assignments and take time to rest.)

But despite the setbacks, I had a lot in my favor. My will to succeed was very powerful. I really wanted to feel better and I wanted to get along better with loved ones. So I stayed on my kick-sugar path, all the while creating foolproof tools and techniques, which you'll learn shortly.

Soon, Connie the Sad Sugar Sufferer vanished. Within weeks, *all* 44 of my symptoms disappeared! After years of "failing," I finally broke free of my sugar addiction.

Within weeks, I became more energetic, happier, exuberant, and just plain glad to be alive. And I grew increasingly *astonished* that just that one simple change of quitting sweets and quickie carbs could make me feel so good. My transformation was nothing short of extraordinary!

My dark, depressing brain fog, overpowering exhaustion, and self-disgust disappeared. My PMS lessened by about 95 percent. The heavy, horrible burden that had been dragging me down lifted. Instead, I was infused with an exhilarating feeling of freedom and pride. My weight soon normalized, too, and I became trimmer and slimmer. I started working out enthusiastically. And sooner than you'd expect, I didn't crave sugar anymore. Amazing!

After shedding my sugar habit, I felt a newfound admiration and appreciation for my body, and I became determined to treat my living temple with the respect and reverence it deserved—quite an unusual feeling for me. I began savoring slow, alive foods (vegetables, fruits, nuts, seeds, legumes, etc.) instead of quickie, dead, processed foods.

## Meet Some Key Phrases as You Break Free, Too

Before we go any further, let me clarify some terms. When I use the word *sugar,* I'm referring to all sweet, processed nonfoods and sweeteners, including sucrose, dextrose, honey, agave, brown sugar, invert sugar, molasses, maple syrup, raw sugar, high-fructose corn syrup, evaporated cane juice, barley malt, concentrated fruit juice, and maltodextrin.

Meanwhile, I also refer to sugar as *The Sweet White Stuff, The White Stuff* or caloric sweeteners. For that matter, I don't recommend artificial sweeteners, which I consider *Sweet Fakes.* So in this book, you'll learn to dissolve your connection to *all* potentially dangerous sweeteners and find healthier ways to sweeten your foods and life.

You will also want to curtail your intake of processed, white-flour breads, rolls, refined crackers, cereals, bagels, white pasta, white rice, potato chips, and other refined, usually gluten-rich grains. (When I discuss these carbs, I call them quickie carbs, toxic carbs, culprit carbs, much-like-sugar carbs, carb nonfoods, fake foods, nonfoods, killer carbs, fast carbs, unhealthy carbs, risky carbs, quick-fix carbs, or dangerous carbs.) *All overly processed carbs* are speedily metabolized in our bodies in a manner that's similar to sugar, which is why they can be *just as dangerous.* In other words, a slice of cake, a piece of white bread, a portion of white rice, or, for that matter, a white potato will all spike your blood-sugar levels.

cont. on next page

Please note also that my choice of the phrases *The Sweet White Stuff* and *The White Stuff* is deliberate. As the late William Dufty declared in his landmark, best-selling 1975 book, *Sugar Blues*, "the difference between sugar addiction and narcotic addiction is largely one of degree."

He goes on to explain: "After all, heroin is nothing but a chemical. They take the juice of the poppy and they refine it into opium and then they refine it to morphine and finally to heroin.

"Sugar is [also] nothing but a chemical," Dufty continued. "They take the juice of the cane or the beet, and they refine it to molasses and then they refine it to brown sugar and finally to strange white crystals."

The bottom line is that over-consuming both sweets and fast carbs can dramatically cut short your life. Soon, you'll find out more about the link between quickie carbs and what I call *The Preventable Big Killers*—heart disease, cancer, type 2 diabetes, and obesity.

What's more, I began to value and appreciate the sweetness of life.

## How I Came to Help People Like You & Create the Sugar Freedom Now Course

In 2001, three years after I quit sugar, I began researching and writing my book *Sugar Shock!* One of the first things I did was join support groups for sugar addiction and hypoglycemia to connect with people who were addictd to sugar like I used to be.

By November 2002, I had launched my own nurturing support group online, the free KickSugar on Yahoo, and for the next five years, it quickly grew and thrived while assistant moderators and I helped thousands of people around the globe overcome their sugar addiction by offering encouragement, tips, information, and success stories. Please note that KickSugar is now inactive and has since moved. We're now on Facebook (www.facebook.com/SmartHabitsFans) and on SparkPeople (http://teams.sparkpeople.com/beyondsugarshock).

Almost from the beginning of KickSugar, most members—knowing that I'd been sugar-free for several years—kept asking for specific tools. So I quickly created the 21-Day Kick-Sugar Countdown Program and offered it for free online. Now, more than a decade later, that initial program has matured into my signature, six-week Sugar Freedom Now Course (also called the Break Free of Your Sugar Addiction in 6 Weeks Program).

You can now take my Sugar Freedom Now Course (*www.BreakFreeWithConnie.com*) in three ways—through a live teleseminar/webinar series; self-guided, prerecorded audio course (the easiest and most popular options, which come complete with a private membership site and lots of bonus audio downloads); or at a live weekend playcamp (a fun version of a boot camp) in selected cities.

In all of my programs, I present my road-tested kick-sugar methods and bring in other renowned experts in wellness, weight loss, mindful eating, hypnotherapy, and other areas to teach you valuable skills you can put to use right away.

> **YOU'RE A HAPPY, SUCCESSFUL SUGAR KICKER WHEN . . .**
> You can honestly dish (and face) the dirt about your former bad-girl or bad-boy sugar behavior.

## I Return to School Three Times to Serve You Better

While writing *Sugar Shock!*, I wanted to become better skilled at helping readers like you and my clients (who I coach privately or in groups) attain lasting victory. So first, I attended the Institute for Integrative Nutrition (IIN) to become a certified health coach. While at IIN, I learned over 100 dietary theories and studied with big names in wellness such as Deepak Chopra, M.D., Andrew Weil, M.D., and David Wolfe.

Next, to help clients create effective, empowering, personalized plans to lick their sugar addiction or other bad habits and achieve other life-changing goals, I trained with the Institute for Professional Excellence in Coaching (iPEC) and became a certified professional (life) coach. At iPEC, I discovered many powerful coaching techniques that I now use to help people release their greatness and create an extraordinary, sweeterlicious life.

Finally, because people like you have been begging me for delicious, sugar-free recipes, I've been taking (as I complete this book) cooking classes at the Natural Gourmet Institute for Health & Culinary Arts and other schools.

## Take Heart: You, too, Can Quit Sugar & Get Sweet Redemption

Now that you've learned how going sugar-free has sweetened my life, you may be thinking, *But I'm not like you, Connie. There's no way I could accomplish that!*

Honestly, you can do it, too! Just take a look at the Sweet Success Stories throughout the book. These people are like you, and their lives are far better now than they ever imagined they'd be—all because they broke the spell sugar had on them. If they can do it, why can't you?

# STEPHANIE ZIMMERMAN

## SWEET SUCCESS STORY

### "How I Lost & Kept Off 220 Pounds"

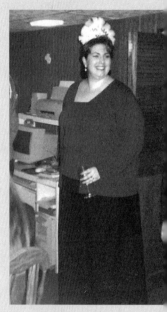

**Hooked on Sugar from an Early Age:** "I've been a sugar addict for as long as I can remember. At age two, I would go into the kitchen in the middle of the night and eat sugar straight from the bowl. Then, in my senior year of high school, I weighed 240 pounds at 5'10½", and kids would holler out, 'Oink, oink! Fat ass!' or 'Hungry, hungry hippo!'"

**Sweets Were the Center of My Life:** "My whole life revolved around food, especially sweets. I always had this *insatiable desire for more*. Baked goods such as donuts and cookies were my biggest downfall. I'd come home with boxes and bags of candy bars, pies, pasta, and chips. Then, I'd close all the blinds, turn on the TV, and eat until I passed out. Eventually, I got up to 370 pounds."

**My Health Was a Mess:** "I became short of breath at the slightest exertion and couldn't climb up a flight of stairs without wheezing heavily. My ankles, legs, and feet were always swollen. I had horrible back pain and achy joints, constant indigestion, and I was always tired. I was also severely depressed, and I was isolating myself from the human race. And I barely made it to work. *All this at age 30!* A heart attack was right around the corner."

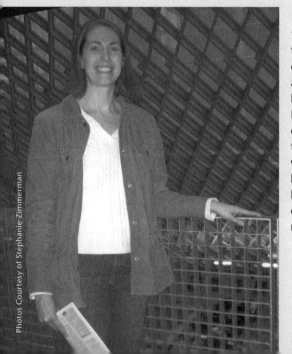

**I'm Now Living the Life of My Dreams:** "Finally, on August 20, 2000, I surrendered to the fact that I'm a food addict, and I stopped consuming sugar, wheat, flour, caffeine, cheese, and alcohol. Without sugar, my body functions like a well-oiled machine. I'm in a job I love; I sing in a band; I see my family often; I have dear friends; I exercise moderately four to five times a week; and I attend support meetings, which help me maintain my recovery. I also have a relationship with God, which I didn't have before, because sugar blocked my spiritual connection. Freedom from sugar addiction is miraculous!"

Photos Courtesy of Stephanie Zimmerman

**I Was Infertile When "On" Sugar, but Now I Have Two Great Girls:** "My period completely stopped from ages 33 to 37. Then, out of the blue, I got pregnant at age 37. I was able to conceive because I let go of the sugar, wheat, and flour. Now, I have two adorable, healthy girls."

**My Relapse Checklist:** "Every night, I do an inventory and check for relapse warning signs, such as eating too fast or in front of the TV; skipping meals; failing to plan my meals; not praying, meditating, or keeping my gratitude list; isolating; and obsessing about food or weight. I encourage anyone who hasn't made out a list like this to do so right away. It is saving my life."

By now, after hearing stories from Stephanie and me, you have a glimmer of and vision for the awesome, amazing, sweeterlicious life that awaits you. But before you begin the simple, six-week plan, it's important to assess, determine, and measure—with a sense of spirit, spunk, and adventure—just how badly hooked you are on sugar or quickie carbs. It's now time for you to take The Sugar Shock Quiz.

## CHAPTER 2

# THE SUGAR SHOCK QUIZ

## FIND OUT HOW HOOKED YOU ARE ON SWEETS & QUICKIE CARBS

**Affirmation: I'm having fun and feeling empowered as I face my Sugar Truth.**

Now, it's time to discover the extent of your sugar addiction. The Sugar Shock Quiz will allow you to explore your feelings about sweets and toxic carbs in a playful, sometimes silly manner, but one that's ultimately serious.

First, let me give you some helpful pointers. As you take this quiz, answer all the questions quickly, because your immediate emotional reactions will give you vital clues as to whether or not you feel "hooked" or even "addicted" to sweets and quickie carbs like millions of people around the world.

At the same time, your rapid-fire answers will help you determine what I call your Sugar Color Code. This is a very simple measuring system, which helps you quickly identify exactly how badly you're hooked and how you might want to quit The Sweet White Stuff—whether cold turkey, gradually, or even allowing yourself occasional indulgences.

Before you begin this quiz, I recommend that you make four copies of it. Here's why: At the end of our six weeks together, you'll take this quiz again. Then, six months from now and a year later, you'll want to revisit it to see how your answers have changed. Of course, eventually your goal is to discover that you're no longer in Sugar Shock and that your favorite sweets no longer have power over you. Let's get going.

1. "If someone ransacked my home, she or he would find candy wrappers hidden behind sofa cushions, a box of cookies stuffed into my closet, or crumbs hanging on to my sweaters and shirts."

    a.  Yes

    b.  No

2. "I really need to lose weight, but I hate how people expect me to just instantly quit my favorite sweet foods and drinks. It's not easy. I've lost track of the number of times I've tried."

    a.  Yes

    b.  No

3. "People find it tough to believe that I have a sugar or carb problem because I'm slim or average weight. But I just can't go one day without my favorite sweets or carbs."

    a.  Yes

    b.  No

4. "I love holidays like Easter, Christmas, Valentine's Day, Thanksgiving, and especially Halloween, because they're great excuses to buy chocolate bunnies, candy canes, gingerbread cookies, chocolate, pecan pie, or big bags of candy."

    a.  Yes

    b.  No

5. "At least one member of my immediate family has had a history of obesity, type 2 diabetes, cancer, or heart disease."

    a.  Yes

    b.  No

**6.** "I've tried many times to lose weight on various diets, but I always fall off the wagon after a while, because I can't stay away from pasta, pancakes, or other processed carbs."

    a.   All the time

    b.   Sometimes

    c.   Rarely

    d.   Never

**7.** "If I had to choose between a night noshing on freshly baked chocolate chip cookies or a romantic evening out with my partner, The Sweet White Stuff would win hands down."

    a.   All the time

    b.   Sometimes

    c.   Rarely

    d.   Never

**8.** "I become quite irrational, lose my cool for no reason, and then take it out on my loved ones."

    a.   All the time

    b.   Sometimes

    c.   Rarely

    d.   Never

**9.** "I often try to hide my sugar addiction. For example, at parties or at home, as soon as no one's watching, I sneak an extra piece of pie, a few extra cookies, or more chips. Sometimes, late at night, I'll even scoop around the ice cream to make it look like I haven't been there."

    a.   All the time

    b.   Sometimes

    c.   Rarely

    d.   Never

10. "My heart sometimes races like a thoroughbred horse in the Kentucky Derby for no apparent reason. It's scary."

    a.  All the time

    b.  Sometimes

    c.  Rarely

    d.  Never

11. "Sometimes I go on crying sprees. I don't know why."

    a.  All the time

    b.  Sometimes

    c.  Rarely

    d.  Never

12. I'm a lethargic lump unless I eat sugary foods, but when I do eat sugar, I become happy and energetic almost immediately.

    a.  All the time

    b.  Sometimes

    c.  Rarely

    d.  Never

13. "I just can't get going in the morning without my sugared coffee, sugary cereal, or a sweet roll. It's a ritual I can't imagine living without."

    a.  All the time

    b.  Sometimes

    c.  Rarely

    d.  Never

**14. "I often get depressed after a sugar high."**

    a.  All the time

    b.  Sometimes

    c.  Rarely

    d.  Never

**15. "I lose all interest in making love to my honey. He/she probably thinks I don't love him/her anymore, but that's not true. I just don't have the desire."**

    a.  All the time

    b.  Sometimes

    c.  Rarely

    d.  Never

**16. "I get the most ferocious, knock-me-down headaches, which make it very difficult for me to function."**

    a.  All the time

    b.  Sometimes

    c.  Rarely

    d.  Never

**17. [Women] "Every month, I have the worst PMS. I become mean, jumpy, irritable, anxious, withdrawn, moody, and depressed. I also get excessive fatigue, lose my sex drive, and find it tough to concentrate."**

**[Men] "My sexual performance isn't as great as it used to be, and I have trouble getting and maintaining an erection."**

    a.  All the time

    b.  Sometimes

    c.  Rarely

    d.  Never

**18.** "As a kid, whenever I cried, my mom or dad would buy me an ice cream cone. Now, whenever I'm depressed, stressed, or frustrated, I reach for ice cream or frozen yogurt."

    a.  All the time

    b.  Sometimes

    c.  Rarely

    d.  Never

**19.** "If I don't grab either a can of soda, candy bar, slice of pizza, or donut by 3 P.M., I turn into a wiped-out zombie."

    a.  All the time

    b.  Sometimes

    c.  Rarely

    d.  Never

**20.** People think that I eat candies, chips, and crackers because I have no will-power. But I know that there's something deeper going on.

    a.  All the time

    b.  Sometimes

    c.  Rarely

    d.  Never

## Are You in Sugar Shock? And Can You Give a Green, Yellow, or Red Light to Sweets?

So, how did you score? Here's how to tally up your results: For questions 1 through 5, give yourself 3 points for "a" and 0 points for "b." For all other questions, use 3 points for "a," 2 points for "b," 1 point for "c," and 0 points for "d."

### 0 TO 20: GREEN SUGAR COLOR CODE
### (YOU CAN GIVE A GREEN LIGHT TO SWEETS.)

Congratulations! It looks like you're not a sugar junkie. You're in complete control. You have the presence of mind and willpower to turn down desserts most of the time, but you allow yourself an occasional sweet. You always have your eye on your health; and for you, balance is a way of life. You probably bought this book for someone else, right?

### 21 TO 40: YELLOW SUGAR COLOR CODE
### (YOU NEED TO BE A CAUTIOUS YELLOW-LIGHTER.)

You have a mild case of Sugar Shock. You need to proceed cautiously around those tempting sweets and quickie carbs, because you can easily forget your best intentions and get overcome by a runaway passion for them, especially if something is upsetting you. Although sometimes you can avert danger, it's a slippery slope fraught with many unpredictable, sweet traps. When you're under stress or duress, for instance, eating even one bite of dessert can have disastrous consequences. Or if you go to a party when you're worried about something, you may keep going back for more cookies or pieces of cake. Your challenge is to tap into your inner calm, strength, and wisdom, and figure out how to stay in control. So ideally, you might want to totally quit or mostly cut sweets before your habit gets out of hand.

### 41 AND UP: RED SUGAR COLOR CODE
### (YOU'RE A RED-LIGHTER. THAT MEANS STOP SWEETS NOW!)

Uh-oh. You have a Red Sugar Color Code. I recommend that you slam on those brakes right now. Sorry to bring you the harsh news, but it's best if you say no to refined sweets and simple carbs totally—at least for now. But take heart, you're among millions of people whose body and brain chemistry won't permit them just one single morsel, because one bite always leads to more—and more and more.

Of course, this isn't a medical diagnosis. But, let's face it, if you're a Red-Lighter around sugar—as many of you are—you're probably in Sugar Shock. This means that your loved ones, friends, neighbors, or co-workers have probably noticed your mood swings, weight gain, difficulty concentrating, and a host of other related symptoms. It's important for you to watch what you eat, because your blood-sugar-related symptoms may already be affecting your quality of life.

Right now, it's probably best if you kick or drastically cut back on your sugar or carb habit immediately before you jeopardize your health, mess up your job, or alienate everyone in your life. In other words, if you're a Red-Lighter, you need to monitor yourself *very, very carefully.* Note, however, that for many people, this realization can be quite liberating.

## Hurrah for You! You're Facing
## Your Sugar and Quickie-Carb Habit

Congratulations! By completing the Sugar Shock Quiz, you've taken a valuable step toward identifying, confronting, and conquering your carb addiction. Now that you know the extent of your challenges, it's time to give you an important Sugar Education 101 so that you learn about some of the severe ramifications of your sugar habit.

## CHAPTER 3

# THE BIG PREVENTABLE KILLERS

## YOUR SWEET TOOTH CAN KILL YOU

**Affirmation: I'm ready to quit toxic carbs
now that I know how dangerous they are.**

It's now time to explore the many alarming health hazards that may be in store if you stay on your Sugar Shock roller-coaster ride. My goal in this chapter is to scare the living daylights out of you, which will, in turn, catapult you into taking positive, sugar-spurning action—and fast!

That's why my tone in this chapter is quite different. I won't be the warm, friendly, compassionate Connie you'll find in the rest of this book. I'll be blunt as I brutally dish the sour truth about sweets.

For your sake, I'll also come down hard on you, much as my doctor did with me when he ordered me to (in so many words): "Kick sugar now or die young."

So I'll get right to the point. *Your sugar habit can kill you well before your time.*

If you continue to play Sugar Shock roulette by overdosing on your favorite sweets and quickie carbs such as pasta, French fries, and white rice, as well as soda, juice, and energy drinks, you could be headed—if you're not there already—on a path to obesity and serious, life-threatening diseases.

## The Big Preventable Killers

More specifically, your habit of splurging on sweets can trigger what I call The Big Preventable Killers, which lead to some of the highest mortality rates.

## The Big Preventable Killers

Coronary Heart Disease
Cancer
Stroke
Type 2 Diabetes and Related Kidney Failure
Alzheimer's Disease

In all, your sugar habit can cause and/or aggravate nearly 150 serious health problems, including fatigue, osteoporosis, arthritis, Crohn's disease, migraines, emphysema, kidney disease, memory loss, food allergies, asthma, gallstones, cataracts, sexual dysfunction, gout, depression, and even infertility. Sugar can also speed up the aging process. If the dangers I now spell out for you don't scare you into action, then at least let me appeal to your vanity: if you hang onto your habit, you'll look older than you really are.

For decades, leading researchers, journalists, and respected experts have been warning you about the perils of sugar and refined carbs. Important stories have appeared in top TV news shows and major newspapers and magazines. Despite all that, much of America still remains in the dark about the potentially deadly dangers of both sugars and processed carbs.

## How Sugar and Quickie Carbs Throw
## Your Body into Crisis & Make You Fat & Sick

It's important for you to understand how your habitual sugar and toxic carb practices can wreak havoc on your body, causing weight gain and serious medical problems.

Here's what happens: Normally, when you eat sugary food and carbohydrates (even complex ones), your body's digestive system breaks the food down into glucose, a simple sugar that is your body's main source of energy. Glucose is easily absorbed into your bloodstream. When your blood glucose (also known as blood sugar) rises, that's a signal to your pancreas to release insulin, which regulates your body's blood-sugar levels and escorts glucose into your cells, where it's used to create energy.

Now, when you mindlessly keep noshing on potato chips and drinking soda all day long, your body produces excess glucose (anything you don't need immediately for energy), which is first converted into glycogen, the storage form of glucose.

Your body can only store a limited amount of glycogen, so excess glucose is stored as body fat.

"People get fat because they eat all these carbs, and sugar makes everything worse," explains science journalist Gary Taubes, author of the bestseller, *Why We Get Fat: And What to Do About It.* "Once your liver and your lean tissue become resistant to the hormone insulin, your pancreas will respond by secreting more insulin. And when we start to become insulin resistant, all carbs then work to make us fatter than we should be. It's all regulated through insulin," Taubes adds, speaking on my *Gab with the Gurus Radio Show.*

Ultimately, releasing all that excess insulin can cause huge health problems for you, Taubes explains. For instance, after you eat so many desserts and much-like-sugar carbs (like white rolls, mashed potatoes, and pasta), too much insulin in your blood can trigger low blood sugar or hypoglycemic reactions such as difficulty concentrating, low energy, or even mood swings. Many of you probably have been experiencing these highs and lows for years, as I once did.

Meanwhile, those of you with type 2 diabetes can have both high blood glucose *and* high insulin levels when you eat sugary carbs, because you may have insulin resistance. Your cells aren't letting insulin and glucose in. This deadly combination can contribute to heart disease; cancer; eye, kidney, and nerve damage; and more than 100 other health hazards.

☆ ☆ ☆ ☆ ☆

## Five Stars to "America's Doctor": Dr. Oz Blows the Lid off Sugar's Deadly Dangers

Millions of Americans are becoming sugar conscious, thanks to renowned cardiac surgeon and Emmy Award winner Dr. Mehmet Oz. In fact, just as I was writing this chapter, *The Dr. Oz Show* ran a phenomenal segment, "The #1 Food Dr. Oz Wants Out of Your House," in which he named sugar #1 on his most wanted list.

In the episode, Dr. Oz—along with researcher Miriam Vos, M.D., from Emory University, and pediatrician Alan Greene, M.D., author of *Feeding Baby Green*—explained how eating too much sugar can put you at major risk for high blood pressure, high cholesterol, liver disease, and insulin resistance.

Viewers were shown how excess sugar becomes mushy, gross goop in your bloodstream. Dr. Oz used a shredder to show you how your liver breaks down sugar. An audience member helped Dr. Oz mix bits of red paper (representing sugar) with a thick clear liquid to show how all that sugar becomes globs of fatty triglycerides—the stuff that clogs up your arteries and causes heart disease, and builds up in your liver to cause nonalcoholic fatty liver.

So, let's give a big round of applause to the pioneering Dr. Oz, who is educating—while entertaining—millions of Americans to become sugar-wise. Because of his exemplary work, Dr. Oz gets the *Beyond Sugar Shock* Five-Star Award for being a Sugar-Education Crusader.

In other words, as Taubes concludes, *"sugar is very likely toxic."*

At this point, you can figure out why I've come up with one of my favorite phrases, *toxic carbs*. Now, let's delve into the connection between sugar and heart disease.

## Sugar Increases Your Risk for Heart Disease & Other Heart-Health Problems

Although you may worry that eating too much *fat* contributes to heart disease, by and large, people almost always completely overlook another more damaging offender—sugar.

That's right. The Sweet Stuff can cause heart disease far more quickly than fat or cholesterol ever can. That's why it's *more* important to carefully monitor your sugar intake than the amount of fat you consume. If you're surprised, you're in good company. Whenever I give lectures and workshops, people are astounded by this fact.

Cardiologist Stephen T. Sinatra, M.D., medical consultant for my book *Sugar Shock!* insists that *"the #1 cause of the hardening of the blood vessels is excess insulin"* and not fat, as many of you may believe. *"The most effective way* to prevent coronary disease is to keep your insulin levels down," he says. In other words, eat fewer sweets and much-like-sugar carbs to protect your heart.

Groundbreaking research now confirms sugar's pivotal connection to your heart health. For instance, one landmark medical study, from Emory University's School of Medicine in Atlanta, which was published in the prestigious *Journal of the American Medical Association*, found that people who consumed the most added sugars were *more likely* (than people who eat less or no added sugars) to have higher cardiovascular disease risk factors, including higher triglycerides, and higher ratios of triglycerides to HCL or the "good" cholesterol. (Triglycerides are the major form of fat stored in our bodies, and elevated triglyceride levels are considered a risk factor for arteriosclerosis or hardening of the arteries, the leading cause of heart attacks.)

The study's lead author, Miriam Vos, M.D., concluded that "the more added sugar, the worse [your] cardiovascular disease risk."

In other words, you may be headed for a heart attack if you're consuming 21 or more teaspoons of added sugars per day, which Dr. Vos cites as the average amount per person.

Please note, however, that I and other experts believe many of you consume *far more*—perhaps 50 teaspoons (or a little more than one cup) of sugar daily.

What this means is that you may be getting between *20 percent to one-third of your calories—if not more—from sugar* and other sweeteners such as evaporated cane juice, dextrose, high-fructose corn syrup, crystalline fructose, honey, agave, and others, which you find in prepared foodstuffs.

The fact remains: Whether you're having 21 teaspoons or 50 teaspoons of added sugars or sweeteners, you're *overdosing* on these legal substances—and putting yourself at risk for heart challenges. But the good news is that when you decrease your sugar intake to five or six teaspoons per day or less, you can lower your heart disease risk.

## Just How Much Sugar Is too Much for You?

Private clients, guests at my lectures, or attendees of my Sugar Freedom Now Course often ask me: "I know that I need to cut back on sugar. But, Connie, just how much sugar is okay to consume every day before it can damage my health?"

Let me set the record straight. Sure, in an ideal world, you'd consume no or very little added sugar. But, let's face it, for many of you, that's not realistic. After all, sugar in its many forms is pervasive in our food supply, and it's often "hidden" in processed foods found in jars, cans, boxes, or packages.

So to answer your question, I recommend that you follow the figures cited by Dr. Vos, who found that people with the best cardiovascular health consume only

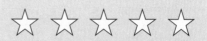

## It Warms Our Hearts: The American Heart Association Takes the Lead!

Americans' staggering sugar consumption became of such concern to the American Heart Association that, in August 2009, the organization spoke out against added sugars for the first time. Many health experts and I heartily applauded the AHA's bold stand.

In a landmark scientific statement, published in *Circulation: Journal of the American Heart Association*, the AHA asserted that high intake of added sugars is implicated in many health conditions, including obesity, high blood pressure, high triglyceride levels, inflammation, stroke, and other risk factors for heart disease.

The AHA statement notes that *added sugars*—as opposed to *naturally occurring sugars*, which you find in vegetables, nuts, legumes, and fruits—along with alcoholic beverages, should provide only "discretionary calories." That means you should only consume them sparingly.

Furthermore, the AHA pointed out that soft drinks and other sugar-sweetened beverages are the number one source of added sugars in the American diet.

"Sugar has no nutritional value other than to provide calories," University of Vermont associate provost and nutrition professor Rachel K. Johnson, Ph.D., lead author of the AHA statement observed.

"Consuming foods and beverages with excessive amounts of added sugars displaces more nutritious foods and beverages for many people."

*cont. on next page*

*cont. from previous page*

☆ ☆ ☆ ☆ ☆

The AHA recommends that most American women consume no more than 100 calories and about 25 grams (about six teaspoons) of added sugars per day. Men, the organization asserted, would be wise to consume no more than 150 calories and about 37.5 grams (or nine teaspoons).

In addition, the AHA also suggests eating a diet rich in fruits, vegetables, high-fiber whole grains, lean meat, poultry, and fish, as well as low-fat dairy products, and it urges people to make sure that foods high in added sugars are *not* taking the place of foods with essential nutrients, or increasing their total calorie intake.

Because the forward-thinking American Heart Association is taking the lead against excess added sugars, it gets the *Beyond Sugar Shock* Five-Star Award for being a Sugar-Education Crusader.

five or six teaspoons of sugar—or less—each day.

In fact, my mentor, colleague, and friend Nancy Appleton, Ph.D.—a clinical nutritionist and one of the preeminent sugar experts in the country—maintains that most healthy people can handle *only about two teaspoons of added sugar at any one time,* two or three times a day. That also comes to *six teaspoons total* per day.

More than three teaspoons of refined sugars at a time, she says, will "throw your body out of balance, suppress your immune system, and attack your body like a foreign invader."

But, adds Dr. Appleton—who's been studying sugar's dangers since the 1970s—"consuming *any simple sugars,* including concentrated fruit juice, honey, maple syrup, rice syrup, and agave, etc., can *seriously* compromise your health."

This brings us to another very important observation. You simply don't *need* added sugars to survive. That's because you can get plenty of glucose—which your brain and body need to function—from vegetables, fruits, nuts, seeds, and whole grains.

Now, I'm not giving you carte blanche to eat two teaspoons of sugar three times a day. If you have prediabetes, type 2 diabetes, heart disease, obesity, hypoglycemia, or cancer, you'd be wise to stay away *totally* from sugar and refined carbs. (Of course, you should speak with your physician, who can give you specific dietary advice.)

After thinking about this for many years, I've come up with what I consider a happy middle ground. If you do *not* have medical reasons to avoid sugar, then you may give yourself permission to have four bites of sweets once or maybe twice a week. Of course, this plan goes out the door if you found that you're a Red-Lighter in the Sugar Shock Quiz. In that case, I suggest you proceed with extreme caution and go cold turkey.

## Another Big Killer: Cancer Feeds on Sugar

These days, just about everyone shrinks in fear when one word is uttered— *cancer*. While we often hear that cancer may be linked to smoking, asbestos, pollution, pesticides, sun exposure, or red meat, one of the best-kept secrets is that sugar fuels the growth of cancer.

Don't believe me? Consider a few studies. Researchers from the State University of New York at Buffalo found that women with high blood-sugar levels had a higher risk of developing breast cancer. They also discovered that females with the lowest blood-sugar levels at the beginning of the study had about one-third the risk of developing breast cancer compared to those with the highest levels of blood sugar.

More researchers from the University of Minnesota's School of Public Health found that drinking two or more soft drinks per week increased the risk of developing pancreatic cancer *nearly twofold*, compared to individuals who consumed no or very few sugar-sweetened beverages. Although pancreatic cancer is one of the more rare cancers, it is one of the most lethal, with only 4 percent of those diagnosed still alive five years later. And sugar can only aggravate your condition.

Now for more scary news. Scientists from the University of Utah discovered that younger men with the highest intake of sucrose (table sugar) had a 60 percent greater risk for colon cancer than people who ate the lowest amount. This study also found that those most susceptible to developing this cancer had a low fiber intake, were sedentary, and overweight or obese.

Clearly, we cannot ignore this frightening cancer-sugar connection, and one of my goals is to wake you up to this phenomenon. It just might save your life or that of a loved one.

## How Does Sugar Promote Cancer?

While it's true that the sugar-cancer connection is not as direct as, say, smoking cigarettes and getting lung cancer, the underlying biology is just as insidious. As I've explained, recent research reveals that high blood-sugar levels are associated with increased risk for several types of cancer. We also know that obesity is linked with hormonal changes that can fuel cancer growth.

Our bodies can detect and destroy most abnormal cells, but if cancerous cells take root, they can easily grow and spread, especially if you "rev them up" by eating lots of sugar.

Bear in mind that all your cells need glucose (blood sugar), but cancer cells are "glucose guzzlers," contends Keith I. Block, M.D., author of *Life Over Cancer* and a renowned integrative cancer-care specialist and medical director of the Block Center for Integrative Cancer Treatment. "In other words," he says, "most cancer cells thrive on a high sugar diet . . . if you strangulate the supply of sugar to the tumor, it may actually trigger a form of *biological suicide among the malignant cells* . . . very few cancers can survive without a steady supply of glucose."

Indeed, the good news then is that just as excess sugar provides an ideal climate for cancer to grow, when you cut out those toxic sweets and carbs, the lack of sugar offers an unfriendly environment to this foreign invader, so the cancer cells will not thrive.

The bottom line: if you have cancer or are at risk of getting it—because of your sugar habit, family history, lifestyle, etc.—you'd be wise to make a plan to get off sweets and refined carbs *now,* not next week.

## The Fructose Shock Connection: Are Processed Foods Making You Fat?

Now, let's talk about how eating too many processed foods may be the reason why you're consuming so much sugar.

First, look at the facts: most major food manufacturers began replacing sugar (made from sugar cane or beets) with the less expensive high-fructose corn syrup in the 1970s and 1980s. They started adding it to thousands of processed foods and beverages, including soda, breads, crackers, cereals, yogurt, ketchup, and mayonnaise, as well as frozen and fast foods. At around the same time—as consumption of HFCS soared—obesity rates in the U.S. skyrocketed. According to the Centers for Disease Control and Prevention, in 1970, around 30 percent of the U.S. population was overweight and 15 percent was obese. Today, more than two-thirds of Americans are considered overweight or obese.

Each year, the average American may be consuming as much as 103 pounds of refined fructose, including high-fructose corn syrup, according to food scientist Russ Bianchi, managing director and CEO of Adept Solutions, Inc., a global food and beverage product development firm. Please note that I'm *not* citing official USDA figures of about 79 pounds per person, which are "grossly underreported," according to Bianchi.

All this additional fructose has led researchers to study the sweetener's impact. In fact, research from Princeton University showed that fructose can make you fat faster than other sweeteners. Scientists there discovered that rats with access to a high-fructose corn syrup solution gained *significantly more weight* than those offered table sugar—even when their overall caloric intake was identical.

During an interview with Bartley G. Hoebel, Ph.D., renowned Princeton University addiction researcher and psychology professor, he explained to me that "Some people have claimed that high-fructose corn syrup is no different than other sweeteners when it comes to weight gain and obesity, but our results make it clear that this just isn't true. When rats drink high-fructose corn syrup at levels well below those in soda pop, they become obese—every single one, across the board. Even when rats are fed a high-fat diet, you don't see this,"

Some experts now believe that your body doesn't metabolize fructose in the same way that it processes other sugars. The theory goes like this: when fructose enters a cell, enzymes break it down, but then the actions of these enzymes raise blood pressure, increase blood levels of artery-clogging fat, and eventually cause obesity.

Researcher Richard J. Johnson, M.D., who has conducted extensive studies on fructose's effects on our health, concludes that "chronic consumption of foods sweetened with fructose seems to promote biochemical changes that prevent the brain from receiving messages from appetite hormones—even when you are not consuming fructose."

"This fructose phenomenon leads to "substantial weight gain in animals," he observes. "Studies suggest that the same thing occurs in humans who consume too much fructose," explains Dr. Johnson, co-author of *The Sugar Fix: The High-Fructose Fallout That Is Making You Fat and Sick*, and professor of medicine and chief of renal diseases and hypertension at the University of Colorado.

If you're a big fan of processed foods and overweight or obese, this information may help explain why it's been such a struggle for you to get rid of your excess pounds—and keep them off.

## Soda Drinkers, Beware: Your Habit Leads to Weight Gain, Type 2 Diabetes, & More

If you're consuming two or more soft drinks a day, you're also setting yourself up for a variety of health hazards. Indeed, several studies now show that long-term consumption of sweetened beverages such as sodas, teas, and fruit juice drinks, or cocktails—which are almost always sweetened with high-fructose corn syrup—contributes to weight gain, high blood pressure, metabolic syndrome, type 2 diabetes, and kidney disease.

As you may already know, soft drinks are the #1 source of added sweeteners. Indeed, the Center for Science in the Public Interest (CSPI) came up with an apt term for soda—*liquid candy.* If you think diet sodas are a safer alternative, you need to be aware that artificially sweetened drinks can also cause you to pack on the pounds—researchers dub this phenomenon "paradoxical weight gain." You'll discover more about this later.

Just how much soda are we guzzling? In 2009, the average American drank 543 eight-ounce servings per year. The U.S. has the highest per capita consumption of carbonated soft drinks in the world, according to *Beverage Digest.* All this soda is taking a huge toll on our health. Here are a few findings:

- *Weight gain:* The relationship between soft drink consumption and body weight is so strong that researchers at the Harvard School of Public Health and other institutions calculated that for each additional soft drink consumed, the risk of obesity increases 1.6 times among children.

- *Obesity and related health issues:* Drinking one or more soft drinks per day (whether diet or regular soda) was correlated with a 31 percent higher risk of becoming obese, as well as a 30 percent higher chance of increased waist circumference, and a 25 percent greater chance of having increased blood triglycerides or fasting hyperglycemia (high blood sugar above 100), according to a study in *Circulation,* the journal of the American Heart Association.

- *Type 2 diabetes:* People who consumed one to two sugary drinks per day (versus none or less than one per month) increased the risk of type 2 diabetes by 26 percent and the risk of metabolic syndrome (a precursor to cardiovascular disease and diabetes) by 20 percent, according to researchers from the Harvard School of Public Health and other institutions, who did a meta-analysis (which combines the results of multiple studies) of 11 studies.

- *Bone fractures and osteoporosis:* Studies also have linked soft drink consumption with lower bone mass and increased fractures, especially in teenage girls. One study, published in the *Archives of Pediatrics &*

*Adolescent Medicine*, concluded that girls who drank soda had *three times* the number of fractures as girls who didn't. Among active girls, cola beverages increased the fracture rate *five times*. In addition, soda drinkers have worse overall diets, too.

If you drink a lot of soda, I recommend that you consider switching to sparkling water or sugar-free seltzer so you can still enjoy that refreshing bubbly sensation. But check the label, though, to make sure no sweeteners have been added.

## Another Big Killer: Your Sugar Habit Also Can Lead to Type 2 Diabetes

Curiously, whenever people are diagnosed with type 2 diabetes, their doctors may not recommend quitting sugar. Instead, chances are good that their doctors will tell them that it's fine to consume sugar *in moderation*. In fact, whenever they first come to me for help, new coaching clients with prediabetes or type 2 diabetes *almost always* tell me that it was *their* idea and decision to quit sugar and most quickie carbs—not their doctors' recommendations. That's why it's important for you to find a doctor who "gets it"—meaning that he or she understands the connection between excessive sugar intake and developing type 2 diabetes.

## The Other Risky Whites

Sugar and white-flour foods aren't the only white foods that can harm you. In fact, they're part of what I call The Other Risky Whites, which form a substantial part of the S.A.D. Here's a quick preview:

**Salt:** About 150,000 people die prematurely each year because of their salt habit. While you need a small amount of sodium for your health, the typical American consumes so much that it is a primary cause of high blood pressure (hypertension), which is a major risk factor for heart disease and stroke. Unfortunately, many restaurants and fast-food places overuse salt to make their foods taste better.

**Artificial Sweeteners:** About 194 million Americans consumed low-calorie, sugar-free foods and beverages in 2010, up from 78 million in 1986. As noted previously, consuming these Sweet Fakes may lead to weight gain.

**Dairy Products:** About 75 percent of people around the world are lactose intolerant, according to the Physicians Committee for Responsible Medicine. Some 30 million to 50 million Americans experience intestinal discomfort after consuming dairy products, with symptoms such as nausea, stomach cramps, bloating, gas, or diarrhea.

**Gluten (Wheat and Many Other Grains):** Once thought rare, about 3 million Americans (or 1 in 100) now suffer from celiac disease, according to the Mayo Clinic. Celiac disease is the most common genetic disease of mankind, but only 1 in 4,700 cases is ever diagnosed. Meanwhile, millions more have gluten sensitivities. You'll get more information about this shortly.

Diabetes is now the seventh leading cause of death in the United States, which contributes to deaths from heart disease, kidney disease, and cancer. Meanwhile, the epidemic is expected to get much worse—the CDC projected that as many as one in three adults could have diabetes by 2050 if current trends continue.

About 23.2 to 24.5 million Americans had type 2 diabetes at the time this book went to print. In addition, 79 million adults had prediabetes, which is a condition in which blood-sugar levels are higher than normal, but not high enough to be diagnosed as diabetes.

## Research Pours In Confirming the Sugar–Type 2 Diabetes Link

**YOU'RE A HAPPY, SUCCESSFUL SUGAR KICKER WHEN . . .**
You ravenously read about sugar's dangers, because you know that the more you get shocked, the more motivated you will be to let go of your addiction.

In recent years, a growing number of medical studies have found a pivotal connection between eating too many sweets and getting type 2 diabetes.

"The overall amount of fat in the diet is not the problem," says preeminent Harvard University researcher, physician and nutritionist Walter Willett, M.D., Dr.PH, who has conducted a number of groundbreaking nutrition studies that explore this issue.

Indeed, those excess carbs, not fat, are to blame for various diseases. "If Americans could eliminate sugary beverages, potatoes, white bread, pasta, white rice, and sugary snacks, we could wipe out many of the problems we have with weight, type 2 diabetes, and other metabolic diseases," Dr. Willett told me via e-mail. He says avoiding unhealthy carbohydrates is an important part of that solution.

"The findings are consistent. A high-glycemic diet is consistently related to type 2 diabetes," adds Dr. Willett, who was citing research that began in 1976 with the landmark Nurses' Health Study and now includes data on 238,000 participants.

This much-cited research really nails down just how related type 2 diabetes is to your lifestyle, because the nurses who developed the disease were consistently overweight, didn't exercise, and ate ample amounts of sweets and refined carbohydrates. (What you may find remarkable—as I do—is that the study participants were nurses, whose mission is to heal you.)

After watching those nurses for three-plus decades, the scientists found that those "with a higher intake of refined starches and sugars had approximately *twice* the risk of developing type 2 diabetes, compared to those with a low intake of these quickie-carb foods."

In addition, a meta-analysis, also from the Harvard School of Public Health, found that regular consumption of soda and other sweetened beverages is associated with a clear and consistently greater risk of type 2 diabetes and metabolic syndrome.

## Quickie Carbs are "Metabolic Bullies" That Make You Fat & Sick

After reviewing the findings of many research studies, the only conclusion that you or I can draw is that sugars and quickie carbs can lead to The Big Killers: heart disease, cancer, type 2 diabetes, and obesity.

Nutritional biochemist Stephen D. Phinney, M.D., Ph.D., who has been studying carbohydrates for more than three decades, has a clever way of damning those much-like-sugar nonfoods.

"Carbohydrates are a metabolic bully," asserts the professor emeritus at the University of California at Davis. What they do is "cut in front of fat as a fuel source and insist on being burned first," explains the co-author of *The New Atkins for a New You: The Ultimate Diet for Shedding Weight and Feeling Great*.

Now, bear in mind that what you don't burn ends up being stored as fat, and your fat won't come out of storage (letting you release weight) as long as you keep eating those quickie carbs. Another important factor to consider is that during the last 30 years, as Americans have been gaining more and more weight, they've also been consuming more and more carbs.

But this book's role is to bring you good news. So take heart: a low-carbohydrate diet can reverse metabolic syndrome and even halt the progression of type 2 diabetes. In fact, in one 12-week study, Dr. Phinney put 40 overweight or obese men and women with metabolic syndrome on a 1,500-calorie diet. Half the participants followed a low-fat, high-carb diet. The other half went on a low-carb, high-fat diet. The low-carb, high-fat participants consumed a total of 100 grams of fat per day, of which 36 grams were saturated. Meanwhile, the low-fat, high-carb group ate 40 grams of fat per day, of which 12 grams were saturated. Fat-phobic readers, get ready to be astounded!

Many of you, I daresay, would be nervous about eating that much fat, right? Well, despite all the saturated fat the low-carb group consumed, at the end of the study, people in the low-carb group had remarkable results—their levels of triglycerides had dropped by 50 percent and their levels of HDL (good) cholesterol increased by 15 percent. Meanwhile, in the low-fat, high-carb group, people's triglycerides dropped by only 20 percent, and there was no change in HDL.

Clearly, this study effectively debunks the fat-can-get-you-fat myth.

## Are You Scared Enough to Take Action?

By now, I hope that you've been shocked and are now motivated to stomp out your toxic-carb ways. If you're still on the fence about whether or not to take the no-sugar plunge, then dig up more dirt about carbs' dangers. Just see the Recommended Reading List on my Sugar Shock Blog or Beyond Sugar Shock website.

But I'll assume that you're scared enough to take positive steps to achieve good health. Now, before you embark on this program, let's take a look at how you got addicted in the first place. You'll also find out about The Five Stages of Sugar Bondage (some or all of which you'll travel through in this book) and The Sweetness Principle.

Please note that, in this next chapter, as you make important realizations, you'll be laying the groundwork so you can hit the ground running.

## CHAPTER 4

# HOW YOU LANDED ON YOUR S.A.D. PATH, THE SWEETNESS PRINCIPLE, AND THE FIVE STAGES OF SUGAR BONDAGE

**Affirmation: I feel relieved now that I know how I got hooked on sugar.**

Before you begin your six-week adventure to overhaul your negative mind-set, establish smart habits, and begin your sweeterlicious new life, I want to reassure you that even if you're not yet fully committed to giving up (or significantly reducing your intake of) The Sweet White Stuff that you *can* do this.

There's no doubt about it. It can be challenging to part with those seductive sweets, even though you know how harmful they are to your health, relationships, and peace of mind. You may even feel that certain fast-fix sweet snacks possess power over you. Indeed, as many of my coaching clients and members of my Sugar Freedom Now Course have admitted *before* they learn my simple tools, walking away from sugar or refined carbs is, to use their words, "like saying good-bye to a best friend" or "as frustrating as trying to end a toxic relationship."

If you've tried and failed umpteen times to kick your sugar habit, you may have believed that quitting risky carbs was close to impossible—until you picked up this book, of course (smile with me here, please). Right now, you may not even want to *think* about giving up those delectable desserts and their culprit-carb cousins. Your feelings are understandable, reasonable, and even expected. Actually, I'd be surprised if you weren't reluctant to make this powerful, positive change.

It's easy to see why you're overly attached to sweets, quickie carbs, and other S.A.D. junk foods. You might feel like you should take responsibility for everything you put into your belly—and to a certain extent you should—but larger forces are also to blame for why you may be hooked on certain foods.

After coaching many junk-food addicts over the years, I've come to realize that we're all very much alike. We're usually well-meaning, sensitive, caring, giving souls, who have simply veered off track and succumbed to S.A.D. temptations, which bombard and tease us just about everywhere we turn—at the supermarket, mall, corner pharmacy, vending machines where you work, and of course, whenever we watch TV commercials, go online, or pass billboards.

This S.A.D. reality is simply unavoidable. We're incessantly barraged by thousands of societal and environmental cues that drive us to purchase and overeat those cheap, calorie-packed, energy-depleting foods.

Let's face it, though, *food* is far too good a word to use when referring to these processed, packaged *fake foods.* Actually, *New York Times* columnist and best-selling author Mark Bittman dubs them *foodlike products,* and best-selling author Michael Pollan dismisses them as *foodlike substances.* In Pollan's book *Food Rules: An Eater's Manual,* he urges readers to avoid: "anything your great-grandmother wouldn't recognize as food . . . products containing ingredients that a third-grader cannot pronounce . . . [and] products that have some form of sugar or sweetener listed among the top three ingredients."

## The Seductive Sugar-Fat Mix

Undoubtedly, most of you find those sweet, fatty foods the most enticing. In fact, this combination of sugar and fat is what makes fake foods so *palatable.* (That's the buzzword researchers use to signify that something tastes so darn good.)

"Higher sugar, fat, and salt make you want to eat more," one high-level food-industry executive admitted to David A. Kessler, M.D., former U.S. Food and Drug Administration commissioner, as he pointed out in his eye-opening, must-read book *The End of Overeating.*

Of course, companies preparing these processed food concoctions seek to turn a profit. So, backed by extensive market research, they give you what they think you want, what they hope you'll crave, and what they seek to sell. At the same time, food manufacturers engage in clever marketing and labeling to convince you to buy their stripped-down foods.

For instance, aren't you more inclined to purchase packaged foods trumpeted as *low-fat* or *low-calorie* because they seem healthier for you?

But guess what manufacturers add to make these low-fat products taste better? Yes, sugar, carbohydrates, high-fructose corn syrup, and carbohydrate-based fat replacers such as maltodextrin and polydextrose. And if it's a nonfood hailed as *no-* or *low-calorie*, chances are good that chemically created artificial sweeteners are included in the mix, too.

You also may be persuaded to buy cereals touted as *lightly sweetened*. But this just means that the product contains less sugar than its previous version, because the Food and Drug Administration (FDA) doesn't regulate the term. So your lightly frosted wheat-somethings may still be loaded with sugar—even if they're whole wheat. These cereals are often *cookies in disguise*.

## You Call That Natural?

Meanwhile, some of my favorite used-and-abused, unregulated terms are *natural* and *all natural*. I don't know about you, but the word *natural* brings to mind images of Mother Nature's glorious bounty, right? Don't you visualize wholesome, nutritionally rich veggies or fruits that grow on trees or out of the ground? But in our world of 21st-century fake foodstuffs, you can actually get organic and *natural* gummy candy and jelly beans, *natural* licorice, and *all-natural* cheese puffs. Excuse me, but these popped up right out of the ground? Pleeease! To put it bluntly, in the food-label universe, *natural* means diddly-squat.

Can you see how the cards are stacked against you and you're being trained and conditioned like poor Pavlov's dogs to fall prey to the allure of those fake, fast carbs?

### YOU'RE A HAPPY, SUCCESSFUL SUGAR KICKER WHEN . . .
You wonder how you could have eaten all those S.A.D. foods.

### No Matter What Your Weight, You Are Malnourished if You're Eating the S.A.D. Way

It's time to point out an important distinction. When you eat the established S.A.D. way, you are *malnourished*—whether you stand to lose a lot, a few, or even no pounds. In fact, despite what your stomach might be telling you, your feelings of insatiable hunger are for *quality* foods. So when you consume all those sugary carbs, you're neglecting to get enough nutrient-rich vegetables, fruits, beans, quality oils, nuts, seeds, legumes, and whole grains.

More to the point, most people don't even realize the connection between those poor foods they're eating now and how badly they feel or behave later that day, week, year, or decade. When indulging, the typical S.A.D. eater probably thinks more about food's potential impact on her or his waistline, than how repeatedly abusing her or his body with nutritionally bereft foods can trigger a variety of other health woes, too.

## You Get No Lasting Comfort from Comfort Foods

Before we move on, I want you to "get" an important concept, which also may be leading you to use or even abuse quickie carbs. Basically, you crave nutrient-lacking, low-fiber foods and turn to them for relief because you're weighed down by your deep, seemingly never-ending hunger or longing. In short, you often need pacifying—and *now!* But no matter how often you fill your belly with such popular comfort food as donuts, biscuits, mashed potatoes, or greasy chicken wings, you can't ever get *enough*. That's because what you *actually* need is to replenish your Mind, Body, and Spirit with substantive and satisfying emotional, psychological, and spiritual nourishment.

So what exactly are comfort foods? Usually, they're anything but wholesome. They tend to be convenient, often rich, salty, fatty, often fried, usually very processed pseudo foods that you seek to make you feel sentimental, safe, calm, and secure. You look to them to soothe your stress. You may think, *The pancakes that Mom used to make for me are what I need now.* Sound familiar?

Not surprisingly, women's top three comfort foods are ice cream, chocolate, and potato chips, while men prefer steak, casseroles, or soups, according to food researcher Brian Wansink, Ph.D., who polled more than 1,000 respondents.

Contrary to popular belief, however, many turn to comfort foods as a *reward*, not when depressed. In fact, 86 percent of those surveyed reported grabbing comfort foods when they're feeling a happy mood, as opposed to 36 percent, who seek them out when they're blue.

Let's face it, though, there's absolutely no comfort in comfort foods. Instead, as you'll soon learn, those refined S.A.D. foods drive you further and further away from the sweeterliciousness you so crave and closer to disaster, disease, and death.

Later in our adventure, you'll discover how to find comfort in healthy, fun, pleasurable activities rather than those sugary, fatty, processed comfort foods. And by the time our journey together ends, you'll feel like one Sugar Kicker who boldly pronounced, "I've come too far to take orders from a chocolate-chip cookie."

## How This Book Helps You Activate The Sweetness Principle

Let me now introduce you to another powerful, related principle, to which I'll refer in pages to come. There's a pivotal connection between your desire to eat quickie-carb treats or drink sweet beverages and your need for more sweetness in your life. I call this The Sweetness Principle.

I'm talking about almost everything that makes life *juicy*.

Let me give you two personal examples of how I activate The Sweetness Principle in my own life. While researching and writing this book, I became an avid, mesmerized fan of Zumba Fitness, which is an exhilarating, Latin-inspired dance fitness-party. To pursue my passion, I now religiously follow certain favorite instructors who offer classes at Equinox Fitness, my gym, and I've even attended three super-fun Zumbathons benefiting the American Heart Association's Go Red campaign. Every time the catchy music comes on, and we begin our high-intensity, rigorous, sensual boogying to the music, I automatically break into a wide grin. It's so much fun! And after a class, I feel so calm, centered, and *goooood*! (Sugar never gave me that!)

One fellow fan, who seeks out several classes a week and keeps peeling off weight (about 50 pounds so far, at this writing), simply told me, "Zumba makes me happy." Our fanatical love of Zumba epitomizes The Sweetness Principle, which means you find a joyful activity that fills you up, invigorates and uplifts you in a way you never thought possible. (Later, you'll learn more about Zumba and other pleasurable, nonsugary ways to get a natural high.)

Likewise, whenever I hop on my beloved bicycle, put on my helmet and gloves, and start pedaling along a park or river, I'm quickly transported to a serene, soothing, joyful place where I feel connected to the universe. Later, when I'm writing, ideas flow to me without my even trying, and I feel content, recharged, and renewed. Bicycling also helps me tap into The Sweetness Principle. (Later, you'll do an Adventurcise to find activities that make you passionate, too.)

In essence, each of us craves and yearns deep in our bodies, hearts, minds, and souls for that often-elusive, intangible, if not obscure, sweetness. In other words,

# JAMES HAHN II

### "How Lent Inspired Me to Quit Sugar as Penance & Lose 87 Pounds"

**My Rock-Bottom Moment:** "When I was 26 years old, my life was an absolute wreck. At 6 feet tall and 273 pounds, I was obese. Stress, anxiety, terrible heartburn, mild bouts of depression, and sudden outbursts of rage were a daily reality. I had gained and lost nearly 50 pounds four times in eight years, but nothing seemed to stick."

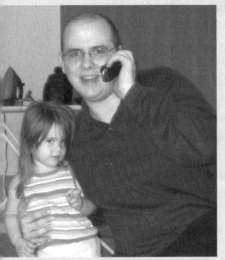

**My Last Horrible Sugar Binge:** "One cold winter night, after another disappointing day at work, I turned to my *two best friends*—cookies and ice cream. I grabbed the biggest spoon I could find—okay, it was a *ladle*—and started devouring the food. After several big bites, self-pity, self-loathing, and self-disgust swept over me. I was doing what I'd promised myself many times never to do again. I just couldn't take it anymore. I began to ask myself, *How many times do you have to go through this? Why can't you change?*"

**Lent Inspired Me to Drop Sugar:** "On January 12, 2006, I decided to kick sugary foods for Lent as penance for my sins. I made it through the 40 days by the grace of God. On Easter Sunday, when I started eating sweets again, the anxiety, depression, and mood swings came rushing back. It was as if a lightbulb went on. I finally realized that sugar is like alcohol for me. I can't stop. If I have one cookie, I'll eat the whole box."

**I'm Happier Than I've Ever Been:** "It's now been more than five years. My moods completely leveled off, my depression vanished, and the everyday anxiety disappeared. I lost 87 pounds. I found and married my amazingly beautiful wife, Jamie, who would have never been attracted to me if I were still obese and hadn't kicked cookies, and we just had our first baby. I also became a certified professional coach, helped my brother lose 126 pounds in eight months, and created a free online community, www.goodlifediet.com, to help others."

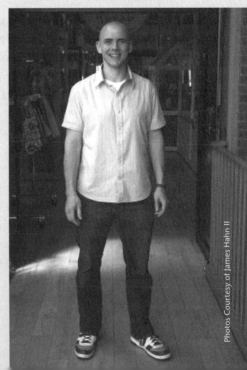

Photos Courtesy of James Hahn II

we're in pursuit of—and often frantic for—a life that's sweeterlicious, which, as I said earlier, stands for sweeter, combined with luscious, delicious, scrumptious, and sensuous. Sweeterlicious also represents fun, joy, passion, pleasure, purpose, harmony, love, laughter, and satisfaction, as well as connection with yourself, other people, and your higher power.

Although Big Food plays a part to addict you, ultimately you've become stuck, trapped, or held captive by your horrible risky-carbs habit, because you're *famished, ravenous, and maybe even desperate* for an abundance of sweeterliciousness.

## The Five Stages of Sugar Bondage: Your Path to Sugar Freedom

Now, it's helpful to learn what I call The Five Stages of Sugar Bondage. After having coached, guided, encouraged, and listened to thousands of sugar addicts around the world for more than a decade and quitting sugar myself, I've observed that *before* you can release your self-destructive carb patterns, you need to pass through these five phases. Only then can you safely land in that delicious place of Sugar Freedom. In other words, giving up your horrible diet is like dealing with periods of grief over a painful loss.

As you learn about the stages, know that you may feel that you're hanging out in several places at the same time or that you're bouncing around between them. Rest assured that your many conflicting emotions, reactions, and frustrations are quite common among people who also seek to escape sugar's stranglehold over them. And remember, throughout this book, I'll be holding your hand to take you gently through the various stages.

## STAGE 1

## Where Most People Are: Trapped in Sugar Denial or S.A.D. Misery

As you learned earlier, the average American is committed—usually for life—to the S.A.D. (Standard American Diet), which is loaded with easily accessible, high-calorie, extensively processed, fiber-stripped, carb nonfoods, unhealthy fats, and, of course, lots of sugar. This is what I call Stage 1 of S.A.D. Bondage or Sugar Bondage.

Most of us remain in S.A.D. denial unless something wakes us up, and we experience a pivotal defining moment.

## STAGE 2

### You Get a Scary or Humiliating Wake-Up Call: Unwanted Flab and Fat, Disease, Disaster, Desperation, Despair, or Disgust Drives You to Seek Help

Usually, to get to Stage 2, something horrible, frightening, awkward, or embarrassing has to happen for carb addicts to escape their challenging rut.

Often, getting that *big wake-up call* is what motivates people to get off the couch and into the gym. Of course, there are exceptions, but in my opinion, carbaholics finally pay intense attention when they get teased or humiliated (for something like breaking a chair); they are disgusted that they can't fit into their size 18 jeans; they are warned by their doctor that their cancer or heart disease can kill them or that their prediabetes will turn into full-blown type 2 diabetes, which means they could ultimately lose a limb or eyesight; they learn that an overweight, sugar-addicted loved one or acquaintance dropped dead of a heart attack; or they are just plain fed up with all the fatigue, anxiety, relationship problems, or emotional challenges that they feel are brought on by their addiction. In other words, for many, it may take being pushed into sour sugar reality.

Despite the hurt or discomfort that this scary Stage 2 time usually gives people, it may be exactly the nudge they need to stop their hemming and hawing, and start acting for their highest good.

## STAGE 3

### You're in the Negative Abyss, and You Alternate Between Anger, Defiance, Resistance, Resentment, Guilt, Self-Blame, Self-Pity, Self-Hate, Self-Criticism, and Why Me? Complaints

Stage 1 of Sugar Bondage could last a lifetime, but a scary wake-up call may suddenly propel you to Stage 2, which generally doesn't last too long. However, Stage 3 could keep you ensnared for years.

In this phase, your emotions may bounce around like a yo-yo, and you may whip yourself into a frenzy of self-blame, self-criticism, and self-hate. At varying times, your feelings of anger, defiance, resistance, resentment, or guilt also come rushing in.

Although Stage 2 can be quite humiliating and scary, Stage 3 can be the most rotten, dreadful, uncomfortable place, as my many coaching clients and I have experienced. In fact, I'm willing to bet that many of you have picked up this book for help to yank yourself out of your Stage 3 abyss, where negativity reigns. During this time, you also may take a woe-is-me stance and behave like a victim. Of course, it takes one to know one—in fact, I once excelled at feeling really sorry for myself.

Over the years, it's been sad, but also fascinating to listen to so many self-pitying gripes, which usually revolve around similar themes. This is when people get into what I call *Why Me? Complaints.*

For instance, the typical grievance goes something like this, *"Why can't I just eat sugar like everyone else?"* Or a sugar addict may grumble, *"It's just not fair!"* Sound familiar?

Since Stage 3 can be tough for many sugar addicts to shake off, later in the program, you'll get many Adventurcises and Playcises that help you glide through this stage rather than stay stuck there for years.


## STAGE 4

### You Feel Insecure, Uncertain, Self-Doubting, Nervous, Scared, and Unsure but also Open-Minded to Your Amazing Possibilities

You hit Stage 4 when you feel insecure, self-doubting, and uncertain that you can even succeed. You're also nervous, scared, and even reluctant about the idea of quitting sugar. Again, these are natural phases and only temporary. In this phase, you're in a pivotal period of transition, because although you may feel apprehensive, unconfident, or indecisive, you're also open-minded. Remember, you'll get Adventurcises later to help you blaze through this phase.

## STAGE 5

### You're on Your Way: Curiosity, Acceptance, Self-Pride, Determination, Confidence, and Commitment

In your final stage of Sugar Bondage, you'll be filled with curiosity, where you'll think something like, *Wow, this sounds like a fun program Connie's outlining.* You'll also be in a stage of acceptance: *Okay, I have this sugar addiction, but I'm finally willing to let it go.* And ultimately you'll reach self-pride: *Yeah, I'm doing it!*

Lastly, you will reach a place of determination: *I'm quitting sugar no matter what!* Then comes excitement: *I'm looking forward to this.*

And finally, you'll be filled with confidence and commitment to your bright future: *Wow, a sweeterlicious life is around the corner!*

So get ready now for exciting times ahead!

After your final stage of Sugar Bondage, you've reached that sublime land of Sugar Freedom. Just bear in mind that this book's six-week program is designed to take you to this final amazing place so you can begin your sweeterlicious life.

### Take a Pledge: It's Time to Commit on Paper

Before you begin your six-week adventure, I recommend that you sign a pledge to undertake it. This will help reinforce your commitment to break away from your unwanted habits and form new ones. Sign your pledge in front of a witness, and share it with a loved one or a therapist. You should also show or e-mail it to a Break-Free Buddy. That's a friend, family member, or even acquaintance, who has the same goal to release a carb addiction. This sugar-free companion will stand by you during your journey and lovingly hold you accountable.

Ideally, your Break-Free Buddy will agree to be there for you by phone or e-mail when you're tempted to slip or if you need some encouragement. If you can't find someone, just visit my SparkPeople group or Facebook (SmartHabitsFans) fan page, and you'll find it easy to connect with people around the world to support you. Now, make three copies of your Beyond Sugar Shock Pledge and place it where you'll see it every day—in a kitchen drawer or your office, attached to your fridge, or near your TV.

Clearly, you now have a lot to consider. So I encourage you to just let the information I shared sink in. Then take the night off so that you're bright-eyed and ready for tomorrow, when you'll begin your six-week Beyond Sugar Shock program.

## PLEDGE to Move Beyond Sugar Shock

I, _____ (name), commit to completing this exciting Beyond Sugar Shock program. I understand that this book will help me evaluate my relationship with sweets and much-like-sugar carbs and create more wholesome, health-promoting habits to lose weight or maintain my ideal weight.

If I find that doing Adventurcises or Playcises in this program brings up unresolved issues and buried emotions, I promise to find appropriate, non-food-related techniques for dealing with them.

Furthermore, I commit to taking special care of myself during the next six weeks. For starters, I promise to begin choosing live, fresh, healthy foods such as vegetables, low-sugar fruits, nuts, seeds, good protein sources, quality fats, and whole grains or dairy products (if I can tolerate them). And I pledge to totally cut out—or at least cut back on—the culprit carbs that have caused me so much harm and sadness. I also agree to find a knowledgeable physician or health-care professional to help support me in this life-changing course.

Finally, I promise to be very gentle with myself as I move forward with this adventure, which could mark the start of a wonderful, healthier life for me as I finally achieve my ideal weight, boost my energy, focus better, accomplish more, get along better with my loved ones, and much more.

(My name)_____

(My signature)_____

(Date) _____

(Witnessed by/optional) _____

# PART II

# YOUR FIRST THREE WEEKS

## GET READY TO SAY GOOD-BYE TO SWEETS AND TOXIC CARBS

## CHAPTER 5

## Week One

# YOUR MIND: FLIP THE SWITCH FROM S.A.D. TO SWEET AND FILL YOUR SWEET ADVENTURE WITH FUN

**I now have a glorious life, and I choose to lean on Sweet, Nonsugary Rewards rather than dangerous sugary foods.**

Woo-Hoo! Today you begin your six-week Beyond Sugar Shock adventure so you can glide toward the glorious, sweeterlicious life you desire and deserve. Soon you'll find that you won't need to rely on those treasured S.A.D. "treats" and culprit carbs anymore. Move over, comfort foods! Bring on sweet, nonsugary rewards instead.

Before we get going, let me share some helpful pointers on how to easily and effortlessly become a rousing, slimmer, vibrant, sugar-free success. First, I urge you to approach the Adventurcises and Playcises in this program—even if they seem unusual—with a childlike curiosity, playful exuberance, and even optimistic glee. Just jump in and allow these simple tips, tools, and tactics to wield their enchanted power over you.

Let's face it, though, your pattern-enforcing sugar- or carb-grabbing routines can be tough to break. That's why I now propose—no, I politely challenge—you to devote the next three weeks to developing new healthy habits, skills, and proactive behaviors. Use the first 21 days of this Break-Free Program to lay the foundation for your better, slimmer, sexier, sweeterlicious life.

You'll warm up, stretch your muscles, and get in shape as if you were training for a marathon, triathlon, or 100 kilometer bike ride. You won't quit sugar in the first three weeks, and you'll even be allowed to politely "sin" with sweets. At the same time, you'll embark on new activities designed to balance your Mind, Body, and Spirit.

In your zeal to escape from your sugar habit and excess flab, many of you may want to skip ahead and ditch sweets and culprit carbs right away. I don't recommend this if you haven't managed to quit sugar by now (unless of course, you are a Red-Lighter or are suffering from a serious medical illness).

Please trust my judgment on this. Rushing in *without a plan* can totally backfire. In fact, many people—when they start working with me—confess that by jumping in without thinking things through first, they quickly slipped back into their old, unproductive sugar and carb routines, even bingeing and gaining more weight than before. My clients and Successful Sugar Kickers have ultimately achieved *more effective, lasting, sweeter success* when they first took time to lay a sweet, solid foundation.

Once you've started implementing fun, healthier habits and embracing the idea that Life is Sweeter Naturally without refined sweets and culprit carbs, you'll be ready to embark on a plan to either totally quit sugar and fast carbs cold turkey or phase them out over time.

You'll also create better eating habits and follow the Beyond Sugar Shock Meal Plan and recipes we provide. Soon, your taste buds will start to change, and you'll discover that wholesome foods are sweeter than you ever remembered.

## Take Weekends Off

To make this program really easy, fun, and manageable, I'm giving you only four main steps per week. You can focus intently and intensely on those four activities for five days. Then, after you've learned and put them into practice, you can give yourself some time to relax, reflect, and allow the information to ease its way into your consciousness.

In other words, I'm inviting you to take weekends off. Don't even pick up this book on a Saturday, unless you really want to. I'm convinced that you'll opt to continue using techniques you've just learned, but you'll be in a vacation-like mode. Just feeling *Hey, I've got the weekends off* will make you even more receptive to your new healthier thoughts and activities.

## Personalize This Plan to Fit Your Needs

The Beyond Sugar Shock program is designed so that you can tailor it to fit your unique needs and personality. You may, for example, want to skip ahead to explore an activity in Week Three. Go for it! Just make sure you go back and complete the exercises in Weeks One and Two, and don't jump ahead to Part III of the book until you've completed your first three weeks.

You also can mix and match menu or snack choices, which are found in the back of the book. Just make sure to watch your portion sizes, and at every snack or meal, select a well-balanced blend of protein, healthy fats, and quality carbs such as vegetables or low-sugar fruits. (Later, you'll get more guidelines on how to eat.)

In other words, do what feels right for you. There's *no wrong way* to experience *Beyond Sugar Shock* as long as you grasp the important principles and try *all* the tools. Before you dismiss a technique out of hand because it seems *too woo-woo* or *too good to be true*, please try doing it at least three times. These exercises really do work, as people around the world have discovered.

Are you ready to win? Let's start your adventure with SWEET, powerful stuff.

## Create a Positive Mind-Set to Kick Sugar

The best way to ensure your success in your Beyond Sugar Shock program is to move forward with a positive, upbeat attitude and, most importantly, maintain that outlook through the weeks to come. So Week One is all about cranking up the volume on your encouraging *I'm doing it now!* voice and embedding positive ideas and suggestions to help you succeed. You'll get powerful, effective ways to retrain your mind so you can *easily and effortlessly let go* of your sugar and carb habits, excess weight, or underlying, self-defeating negativity.

Most people start new eating plans or diets thinking they need huge amounts of willpower. You know how long *that* lasts, right?

Pretty soon, you begin to think *Maybe I can have just a couple of cookies for lunch.* Or, *Oh heck, I've already blown it, so I might as well polish off the entire quart or gallon of ice cream.* Sound familiar?

So we're starting with a mind shift, not a food switch. As you proceed, always bear in mind that you can go one of two ways:

- **S.A.D.:** The toxic, self-defeating, self-doubting chatter in your head that has kept you trapped for years. This is the doomed attitude that prevents you from achieving your goals, both sugar-free and otherwise.

- **SWEET:** The fun, optimistic, energizing perspective. This is the kind of mind-set you want to have to win big.

It's your choice. Yes, it's that simple.
Now here are your four steps for Week One.

Week One: <u>**YOUR MIND**</u>
**STEP 1:** See, Feel & Act As If You've Already Won!
**STEP 2:** Do Sugary Soul Searching
**STEP 3:** Accept Your "-aholic" Nature
**STEP 4:** Team Up with Experts & Seek Support

## STEP 1: See, Feel & Act As If You've Already Won!

### Affirmation: I now see myself sugar-free and feeling great!

Time and time again, people who've accomplished tremendous things have proved that if you believe you'll succeed, it will come to pass. Your goal here is to repeatedly plant positive thoughts in your subconscious mind so that your beliefs will blossom and start coming to fruition.

And you want to dream *big*. "Dream lofty dreams, and as you dream, so shall you become," James Allen urged in his uplifting, perennial classic *As a Man Thinketh*. "Your vision is the promise of what you shall one day be; your ideal is the prophecy of what you shall at last unveil."

Now let the late Napoleon Hill encourage and reassure you: "Whatever the mind of man can conceive and believe, the mind can achieve—regardless of how many times you may have failed in the past, or how lofty your aims and hopes may be."

But just seeing yourself easily passing up on sweets isn't nearly enough.

"You need to *feel* as if you've already ***owned*** that goal," says motivational guru John Assaraf, author of *Having It All* and one of the featured stars in the hit film and book *The Secret*. "You need to believe your new reality more than your current reality," he explained on my *Gab with the Gurus Radio Show*.

Manifestation expert Arielle Ford, author of *The Soulmate Secret: Manifesting the Love of Your Life with the Law of Attraction*, says you need "to *feel* in every cell of your being the outcome you want to create in order to begin to draw it toward you. These *feelingizations* are far more powerful and effective than visualizations [by themselves]. It's the feeling—not the image—that holds the power to attract."

## Affirmation: My Woo-Hoo, Feel-Good Theme Song always makes me feel good.

## Let Music's "Mozart Effect" Work for You

One important way to See, Feel & Act As If You've Already Won is to have fun—yes, lots of it! You want to begin to associate letting go of your sugar and carb habit with deep-seated joy, pleasure, serenity, sensuality, and good times. How? Just let magnificent music work its magic and wipe away your insecure chatter or fear.

Music can soothe you, calm you down, give you confidence, inject you with good cheer, and make you feel strong, hopeful, motivated, and powerful.

Music also can become your reliable, trustworthy, nonjudgmental "companion, spiritual guide, and very immediate friend," explains musician and composer Don Campbell, author of *The Mozart Effect: Tapping the Power of Music to Heal the Body, Strengthen the Mind, and Unlock the Creative Spirit*.

More important, music can help to replace your dangerous S.A.D. carb fixes. Whenever life feels overwhelming or sweets beckon to you, instead of throwing carb caution to the wind, you can lean on this noncaloric, much sweeter, melodic fix.

That's why I highly recommend that wherever you go, bring your iPod or other portable player with you—*especially* if you find it tough to avoid the vending machine at work or the donut store near your home.

In fact, symphonies, choral works, pop songs, and other tunes are so utterly powerful and transformative that the term *Mozart Effect* is now used to refer to a growing body of intriguing research citing the power of music—from composers as diverse as Mozart, Philip Glass, Aqua, and Yanni—to bring about positive emotional, psychological, and physiological changes.

Spending a mere 30 minutes a day listening to "rhythmically homogeneous music" (anything from classical to Celtic to Indian) while doing slow abdominal breathing can actually lower blood pressure, researchers at the University of Milano-Bicocca in Italy discovered.

Your beloved tunes can positively affect your cardiovascular system (expanding the inner lining of your blood vessels and increasing blood flow), according to researchers at the University of Maryland School of Medicine. But when participants in the study listened to music they deemed stressful, their blood vessels narrowed, which reduced their blood flow.

Still more studies have found that listening to or even creating music helps people relieve depression.

### Playcise: Find a Favorite Woo-Hoo, Feel-Good Tune: So Much Better than Sugar!

Now it's time for a fun musical Playcise. Find your own exhilarating, invigorating, inspiring melody that always—no matter what's going on in your life—puts you in an upbeat, optimistic mood, where you're convinced, *I can succeed!*

Your Woo-Hoo, Feel-Good Tune will represent your victorious journey to success, brightness, love, and sweeterliciousness. Your song will lift you up when you're discouraged, invigorate you when you're feeling blah, or give you the motivational boost you need to keep moving toward quality carbs.

Go on a musical treasure hunt. Examine your music library (iPod, CDs, etc.) to find melodies that speak to you. Ask friends, work colleagues, or family members for recommendations. Invite Facebook buddies to suggest ideas. And you can listen to a different, mood-boosting Woo-Hoo, Feel-Good Tune every day on my Facebook page.

I also invite you to visit my Sugar Shock Blog to see my comprehensive list of ideas, which includes links and videos of such inspiring tunes as "Strong Enough" (Cher), "We are the Champions" (Queen), "I'm Alive" (Celine Dion), or "Beautiful Day" (U2). Just go to www.SugarShockBlog.com and click on the header *Find Woo-Hoo, Feel-Good Tunes to Motivate You to Get a Life That Rocks!* Make sure to suggest your favorite melodies, too, so together, we can inspire more people around the world.

## Adventurcise: Pick Your Beyond Sugar Shock Woo-Hoo, Feel-Good Theme Song

List five possibilities for your exhilarating, mood-lifting Woo-Hoo, Feel-Good Theme Song. Pick up-tempo tunes to which you can gleefully dance, work out, or jump around.

1. _____

2. _____

3. _____

4. _____

5. _____

Now, pick your favorite—the one tune that cheers you up every time you listen to it and most symbolizes you winning no matter what.

### My Beyond Sugar Shock Woo-Hoo, Feel-Good Theme Song Is

_____

The runner-up is _____

Why these songs? _____

_____

If you tire of your Woo-Hoo, Feel-Good Tune, just pick another and then another. Keep rotating your selections. You can even alternate from day to day.

## Move to Your Woo-Hoo, Feel-Good Theme Song & Do the Success Strut

It's time to have more fun. First, make sure you're alone. Shut the door and windows. Put on your sneakers and your sexiest workout clothes—something in which you can move comfortably and feel attractive.

Start listening to your Woo-Hoo, Feel-Good Theme Song and crank up the volume—without bothering your neighbors, of course. Next, stand up, breathe deeply three times, feel the song move you, and visualize your Sugar-Free Success. Begin to boogie with glee around your living room. Lean to the right, then to the left. Just move in whatever way inspires you. (If you have weight challenges or injuries, do what you can.)

**YOU'RE A HAPPY, SUCCESSFUL SUGAR KICKER WHEN . . .**
You get a bigger Woo-Hoo from your Feel-Good Tune than you ever got from cookies, chips, or candies.

Now, imagine that you're showering your body with love. While dancing, glide your hands appreciatively, sensuously all over your body—especially parts you like the least. Sway seductively, swivel your hips, and hug yourself.

While the music plays and you dance, gleefully shout "Woo Hoo!" "Yes!" "All Right!" or whatever phrase appeals to you, and raise your arms triumphantly above your head. Feel excitement gushing through your body. Holler with joy that you're *finally* releasing your sugar habit! Yes, you've already succeeded!

As your Woo-Hoo, Feel-Good Theme Song concludes, do the Success Strut. You know what I'm talking about. Hold your head high. Tighten your midsection or core. Smile self-assuredly. Then purposefully stride back and forth across the floor. That's it—confidently strut!

Soon, you'll find that the *instant* you put on your Woo-Hoo, Feel-Good Theme Song, you'll make a joyful association and flip into a victorious frame of mind. Each time you dance to your fun, uplifting tune, you're setting yourself up to succeed.

---

### COACH CONNIE'S SWEET SUCCESS STRATEGY

#### Boogie Often to Your Woo-Hoo, Feel-Good Theme Song!

To get the best results, I heartily recommend that you listen to your Woo-Hoo, Feel-Good Theme Song *at least twice a day*—preferably first thing in the morning (before breakfast) and in the early evening (before dinner). That way, you'll turn to your tune to help you feel good *before* you eat, and you'll be more inclined to make healthy choices. Soon, you'll find that music nourishes you and fills you up in a way sugar never can. Trust me—this works.

---

# MARINA KAMEN (AKA MARINA)

## SWEET SUCCESS STORY

### "How Music Helped Me Shed 100 Pounds"

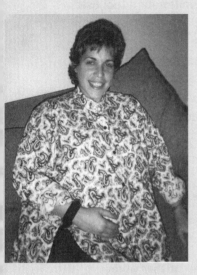

*Note from Connie: Once obese, Marina Kamen (www. MarinaOnline.com) is now a certified fitness trainer, Billboard-charting writer/producer, musician/vocalist, and violinist. Marina—who is known for such inspiring songs as "Today, I Believe," "Strut!" "Dance," and "Never Stop Movin'!"—was a guest on my Gab with the Gurus Radio Show. Here's her story.*

**I Was Always Overweight:** "I was heavy as a child, and my mother was heavy, so I guess there was a little genetics there, but I ate too much bread, too much sugar. I wanted my bonbons, and that put many, many pounds on my bun buns. By the time I was 37 years old, with three children, I had ballooned to 215 pounds, and I have only a 5'3" frame."

**Music Motivated Me to Move & Lose:** "I credit music with motivating me to get off my butt. Being a musician, I started to record, and I began to move and get winded, whether it was walking in place in my house or walking the two miles to work at a good clip. I lost 100 pounds by walking, dancing to my own tracks, and a portion-controlled, well-balanced meal plan."

**My Top Tip—Sneak in Exercise "Snacks" One Minute at a Time:** "Instead of sneaking snacks and junk food when nobody is looking, sneak in some exercise! Stand up and bring your arms over your head, reach over to your sides, and then just hang over and feel the music. Pull in your abdominals, stretch the back of your legs out just for that minute. I do that all day."

**Keep Moving:** "There's just *no better high* than moving as I sing in my tune, 'Never Stop Movin'.' The lyrics are: 'Keep improving. Never stop movin'. Take a good look at what you're doing. Never stop movin'.' So the high that you got from sugar, you should get from movement. It's a better choice, don't you think?"

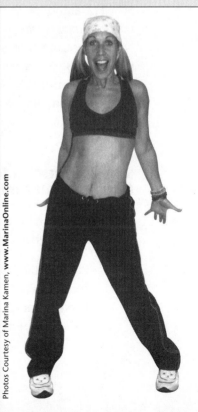

Photos Courtesy of Marina Kamen, www.MarinaOnline.com

## Create a Vision Board of Where You Want to Be

In order to See, Feel & Act As If You've Already Won, you want to envision your beautiful, lean, trim, toned, sugar-free body on a daily basis. In other words, think forward and watch a sexier, slimmer you in *The Now*.

One of the most effective ways to make your weight-loss and sugar-free dreams a reality is to create a vision board. This is a powerful visual manifestation tool used by some of the world's leading thinkers, successful businesspeople, best-selling authors, and now you.

Basically, a vision board helps you harness the law of attraction, a metaphysical belief system that helps you to focus your thoughts and feelings so that they act like a magnet and attract what you want—from health to wealth to relationships. For your purposes, you'll learn to attract a slim, vibrant, healthy body, and a desire for only quality carbs and real foods.

A vision board works because you're both seeing and feeling that you've already achieved your goal. "In effect, it acts like a GPS (Global Positioning System) or visual life-planning program to help you achieve your goals," says Joyce Schwarz, author of *The Vision Board: The Secret to an Extraordinary Life*.

Because our brains are visual, you want to include images on your vision board of what you want your body or life to look like. You're also reprogramming your brain to achieve your desired results.

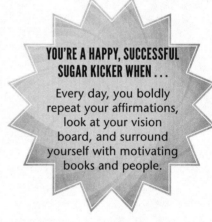

**YOU'RE A HAPPY, SUCCESSFUL SUGAR KICKER WHEN . . .**
Every day, you boldly repeat your affirmations, look at your vision board, and surround yourself with motivating books and people.

## Surround Yourself with Affirmative Notes and Pray

To drive home the fact that you will See, Feel & Act As If You've Already Won, here are some other simple things you can do:

- Post positive notes in prominent places around your home. Some suggestions: "I'm happy without sweets," "I'm at my ideal weight of [xxx] pounds," or "I only desire healthy, nourishing foods that keep me at my perfect weight."

- Keep repeating, with feeling, your favorite affirmation or positive mantra 20, 50, or even 100 times throughout your day. You need to flex your unworked mental muscles.

- Whenever temptation strikes, use an affirmation. Here's one if a candy bar or brownie "calls out" to you: "My cravings pass quickly." Or, "I enjoy eating only healthy, nourishing, real foods." Or, "I'm at my ideal weight."

- If you like, you also can pray in the morning, evening, or in between. Here's a prayer I wrote for you. If this isn't your thing, then skip this.

  Dear God [or Divine Intelligence], please grant me the courage and commitment to release my sugar habit [and/or excess weight]. Please guide me to nourishing foods and beverages. Help me to be happy, healthy, and at my ideal weight of [xxx]. Thank you, God, for this or something much better.

## Motivate with the Masters

One of the best ways to keep on track and stay in a positive frame of mind is to recharge and fill up daily with positive thoughts, motivating quotes, and empowering ideas from motivational experts. For instance, you can rely on some of my favorites—such as *Illuminata* by Marianne Williamson, *You Can Heal Your Life* by Louise Hay, and *How to Get Your Prayers Answered* by Rabbi Irwin Katsof.

**YOU'RE A HAPPY, SUCCESSFUL SUGAR KICKER WHEN . . .**
You ditch the word "lose" when it comes to weight. Instead, you're releasing, dissolving, or simply letting it go.

## Adventurcise: Create "Why I Need to Quit" & Benefits Lists

Removing sugar from your life is a win-win proposition, but it can be tough to remember this when you're tempted by a glazed donut. To help you focus on the long-term benefits of quitting sugar as opposed to the short-term pleasure of taking that first bite, think about why it's absolutely imperative that you let go of your habit.

**Why Do I *Need* to Quit Sugar?**

1. _____

2. _____

3. _____

4. _____

5. _____

**How Will Quitting Sugar Improve My Life?**

1. _____

2. _____

3. _____

4. _____

5. _____

Now make a copy of these lists or put them into your cell phone so they're with you wherever you go. Also, put one in front of your computer and another on your fridge.

## STEP 2: Do Sugary Soul Searching

**Affirmation: Whenever I feel a need to eat something sugary,
I first do Sugary Soul Searching to discover what's eating me.**

Now that you're lifting your Spirits daily with your Woo-Hoo, Feel-Good Theme Song, as well as your Success Strut and Benefits List, I hope you're feeling optimistic, determined, focused, and single-minded.

It's time to go inward and do a powerful process I created that I call *Sugary Soul Searching.* You want to discover dispassionately—without any emotional attachment—how enslaved, ruled, and directed you are by your sugar and carb addiction. Owning up to the reality of your sugar relationship is a potent way to nurture, love, and appreciate yourself, and find the true, magnificent you.

Long-term change won't happen until you find out how you got here. You need to delve deep within to discover what drives you to eat one more donut, candy bar, or slice of pizza. Otherwise, the quickie-carb quicksand can suck you right back in all over again.

The good news is that once you Face Your Sugar Truth, your answers will help you create a road map to help you let go of your demons so you can stop bingeing and release your excess weight for good. And ultimately, when you face *who you are* because of your sugar addiction, you make bold leaps to become *who you can be.*

**YOU'RE A HAPPY, SUCCESSFUL SUGAR KICKER WHEN . . .**
You often focus on the many benefits you'll gain when you go sugar-free.

## Think of Sugary Soul Searching as a Treasure Hunt

It's ideal for you to regard Sugary Soul Searching as something fun, so face your sugar truth with a sense of adventure. Picture yourself as a famous 19th-century explorer who is about to discover a chest of riches. The prize? Good health, stable moods, happiness, better relationships, greater concentration, a svelte body, and much more.

Please be aware that strong emotions may surface. You may get gloomy, remorseful, or upset about how your habit has made you so much less than you can be. However, instead of letting your emotions drag you down, just step outside yourself and calmly, unemotionally observe, without judging, how much you "need" sweets or simple carbs, and how having them affects you. Later, you'll also get some techniques to deal with these powerful emotions. For now, I recommend that you listen to calming, mellow music as you do Sugary Soul Searching. At the same time, you may want to begin keeping a journal to write about your conflicted sugar feelings.

## Adventurcise: Sugary Soul Searching—How Do You Feel About Sweets & Carbs?

**How important is sugar to you?**
_____ Absolutely imperative! How can I live without it?
_____ Very important
_____ Important
_____ Only important when I'm stressed out

**Do you view sugar or simple carbs as a "friend" who will always be there for you?**
Yes _____
No _____
**Why? Write about it in your journal.**

**Or, do you see sugar as a "foe" who will bring you to ruin?**
Yes _____
No _____
**Why?**

**Is sugar both your friend and foe?**
Yes _____
No _____
**Why?**

**Do you feel like an alcoholic or drug addict, who "must" have sweets or simple carbs at certain times—no matter what?**
Yes _____
No _____
**Write why in your journal.**

**I spend _____ ( ___ minutes ___hours) per day thinking, obsessing, or planning my next sugar or carb "fix."**

**Do you overeat large amounts of sweets or high-calorie, processed foods in a short period of time?**
Yes _____
No _____

**When you think about your relationship with sugar or quickie carbs, how do you feel? _____** (Fill in the emotion—sad, angry, depressed, discouraged, disgusted, disappointed in yourself, etc.)

**What weight-loss tricks have you tried?**
Fad diets? Yes _____ No _____
Laxatives? Yes _____ No _____
Self-induced vomiting? Yes _____ No _____
Over-the-counter diet pills? Yes _____ No _____
Overexercising? Yes_____ No_____
Other things? Yes _____ No _____What? _____

If you answered yes to two or more questions, then you may have what many experts consider a food addiction, or your sugar habit may border on an eating disorder. If that's the case, you need to research this further and even seek medical treatment. Let's go deeper now.

## Adventurcise: Sugary Soul Searching—The "I Feel" Process

Now, think about how you're physically and emotionally affected after eating sweets. In other words, after you devour that chocolate croissant, do you get wired and then tired, moody, angry, jittery, anxious, sad, depressed, irrational, confused, negative, and very unlike yourself?

Within one to three hours or even one to three days of eating sugary foods or much-like-sugar carbs, I feel [or I become] . . .

1._____

2._____

3._____

4._____

5._____

**How does this affect your life and your relationships on a daily basis?**

_____

_____

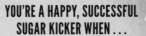

**YOU'RE A HAPPY, SUCCESSFUL SUGAR KICKER WHEN . . .**

You suddenly realize that you haven't thought about sugar for four whole hours!

## Adventurcise: Sugary Soul Searching—Repeat Foods

What foods do you eat again and again? (White bread, soda, sweet rolls, macaroni and cheese, candy bars, ice cream, etc.?) Is your choice connected to a childhood memory? If so, how? Why does this food hold such power over you?

1._____

2._____

3._____

4._____

5._____

## Adventurcise: Sugary Soul Searching—S.A.D. Habits

Do you eat junk foods at certain times of day, such as right after coming home from work, when watching TV, or late at night? Write down what times you're most vulnerable and why.

1._____A.M. Why?_____

2._____A.M. Why?_____

3._____A.M. Why?_____

4._____P.M. Why?_____

5._____P.M. Why?_____

6._____P.M. Why?_____

## How Sugary Soul Searching Helped Me Take the Leap

After my doctor delivered his kick-sugar-now message to me back in 1998, *the last thing* I wanted to do was give up my favorite chewy red licorice, cinnamon hard candies, chocolate-covered peanuts, and quickie-carb crackers. So *the first thing* I did was quiz myself in the manner you're now doing. In fact, Sugary Soul Searching became one of the most pivotal, empowering tactics that I developed and used to overcome my sugar and carb dependence. My coaching clients now love it, too. Just owning up to the fact that we've been hooked allowed us to break sugar's hold over us. This tactic really works!

**YOU'RE A HAPPY, SUCCESSFUL SUGAR KICKER WHEN . . .**

You can't imagine <u>not</u> doing Sugary Soul Searching.

## The Easy 5 W's & 1 H

While quitting sugar in 1998, it hit me that my background as a journalist could offer valuable guidance. As a reporter, whenever you write a story, you always need to answer who, what, when, where, why, and how.

So to unhook myself from my sugar addiction, I began to ask myself these same six journalistic questions any time I felt tempted by sugar or quickie carbs. That soon led to my developing this valuable Sugary Soul Searching tool. Now you, too, can use this powerful process. The next time you're staring down something S.A.D., ask yourself questions using the 5 W's & 1 H:

- *Who* . . . *Who is upsetting me? Who am I with when sweets most call out to me? Who is in control here?*

- *What* . . . *What is upsetting me? What could I do instead of pigging out? What do I really want?*

- *When* . . . *When do I most crave sugar? When (i.e., particular times of day or night) do I most often eat sweets? When will I finally stop the self-destructive pattern?*

- *Where . . . Where am I when I lean on quickie carbs? (In the kitchen, at a fast-food restaurant, in the bakery, in my car, on the way home from work, etc.?)*

- *Why . . . Why am I doing something so destructive? (Why is also significant because you'll know the driving force behind your destructive behavior.)*

- *How . . . How effective is eating sweets? How does this make me feel better? How long will I continue to abuse myself?*

## Dig Deeper to Discover What's Eating You

Imagine that it's been a long, stressful day at work, your boss annoyed you, one of your kids has trampled on your flower beds, your sweetie didn't take out the garbage, you haven't worked out yet, you're late with dinner, and your 14-year-old just brought home a bag of your favorite chocolate chip cookies. *Argh,* right? In other words, you could easily gobble those cookies *before* your child even takes one bite.

**YOU'RE A HAPPY, SUCCESSFUL SUGAR KICKER WHEN . . .**
*What's eating me?* is your favorite question—especially before a bite of a brownie crosses your lips.

The first thing you want to do is ask yourself:

- *What's eating me?* Your reply might go something like this: *I'm angry at my boss, my kid(s), my husband, and nothing is working out right today.*

- *What do I want?* Answer: *Chocolate chip cookies, of course!*

- *Really? Is that what I really, really want?* Answer: *No, not really. What I'd actually like is some "me time" to just chill out.*

- *But what do I really, really, really want?* Answer: *I want my honey to listen to me! And I want more help around the house from my husband and kids.*

- *What else do I want?* Answer: *I want everyone to appreciate me more!*

See what I mean? By asking yourself over and over again, *What's eating me?* and *What do I really want?,* you discover what you *really need*, deep down.

Once you've hit on your truth, instead of bingeing on cookies, you may instead put on some relaxing music, take five minutes to yourself, nicely ask members of your family to help you cut some vegetables or set the table, or dance together to your Woo-Hoo, Feel-Good Tune.

---

### Coach Connie's SWEET Success Strategy

### Befriend Your Worst "Failures"

One of the most valuable ways to liberate yourself from your sugar addiction, excess weight, and negative thinking is to overhaul your concept of so-called failures. Whatever you've allegedly botched up in the past can help you to succeed now. Start regarding your month-long sugar binge, years-long battle with your weight, or carb splurge at lunch yesterday as valuable, instructive, necessary sidesteps or zigzags.

Indeed, your past *slips* are *springboards to victory.* Your so-called failures can become your biggest, indispensable allies, which can set you free for good.

---

### STEP 3: Accept Your "-aholic" Nature

### Affirmation: I now accept my sugar and carb addiction. Because of it, I'm growing.

By now, you probably realize that you may be addicted to The Sweet White Stuff. You may use sugar and quickie carbs to self-medicate, escape from your painful feelings, comfort you, give you a buzz, "fill you up," and help you survive life's unexpected disappointments or hurdles. It's time to Accept Your "-aholic" Nature, as I put it, and come to terms with your junk food addiction.

Think of it this way: because of your addiction, you're becoming a better person. What began as a horrible habit is your ticket to fulfilling your true potential. Pretty cool!

It's also helpful to remind yourself that you're not alone. Most Americans are "problem users" of video games, gambling, sugar, sex, alcohol, or drugs. They're caught in "a never-ending cycle of craving, bingeing, remorse, and withdrawal," says award-winning TV journalist Jane Velez-Mitchell, speaking on my *Gab with the Gurus Radio Show.*

Although many members of the mainstream medical community assert that sugar addiction doesn't exist, a growing body of evidence now suggests otherwise. This wave of new research is so important that the *Journal of Addiction Medicine* has published articles about this "new science" of food addiction. Certain foods, "with sugar the most thoroughly studied," can "hijack" the brain or activate it like drugs, and that "tolerance and withdrawal are exhibited by rats consuming sugar," one article concluded.

In fact, when offered a choice between sugar and cocaine, rats preferred the Sweet Stuff according to scientist Serge H. Ahmed, Ph.D., and colleagues at the University of Bordeaux in France. "The taste of sweetness is much *more rewarding* than *intravenous* cocaine and heroin, even in drug-sensitized animals with a long history of drug self-administration [meaning they'd been hooked for a while]," Dr. Ahmed explained at a food addiction conference.

**YOU'RE A HAPPY, SUCCESSFUL SUGAR KICKER WHEN . . .**
You view your previous so-called failures as your biggest allies.

Wow! Can you imagine? Rats preferred sugar over cocaine and heroin?!

Meanwhile, another study, published in *Archives of General Psychiatry,* by researchers at Yale University's Rudd Center for Food Policy and Obesity showed that in response to a chocolate milkshake, compulsive eaters exhibited similar activity in certain brain regions as people addicted to alcohol or drugs.

I hope this new research reassures you and helps you acknowledge and accept your addiction. By the way, since food addiction research is still pouring in, I invite you to get updates at my Sugar Shock Blog.

# JANE VELEZ-MITCHELL

### Living Without Alcohol or Sugar in an "Addict Nation"

**Surrounded by Alcoholics:** "I grew up in an alcoholic household, so I knew that I drank alcoholically. Things that were cute when I was 18 or 20 weren't so cute when I was hitting my 30s. I was 39 when I finally got sober. But I was very lucky. I never had a DUI or anything, but all addiction leads to incomprehensible demoralization."

**My Rock Bottom Night:** "On the last night I drank, I was doing Snakebites at a party. [These are beer, hard cider, and blackcurrant cordial.] I blacked out, kissed the host, and knocked him down a flight of stairs. They carried me out over somebody's shoulder, and I didn't remember much of it, except in flashes. The next day, I called my friend and said, 'All right, I agree. I have a problem, and I'm going to do something about it.' It's like a shift occurred when I surrendered to my powerlessness over alcohol, and realized, *I don't have to drink today.*"

**I Switched from Alcohol to Food:** "When alcoholics get sober, many immediately dive into sugar. They even serve cookies at recovery meetings. I'd never really cared about food when I was drinking. Then, when I stopped alcohol, food became an issue, because addicts [often] jump from one substance to another. They say we're driving different cars, but we're all headed for the same destination: oblivion. All addictions are about stuffing your feelings, numbing yourself, and escaping pain. If he can't use alcohol, the addict will find something else. So, I started using food."

**Sugar, Evaporated Cane Juice, Agave & Other Sweeteners Became Addictive, Too:** "Sugar [and other sweeteners] started to feel just like alcohol . . . and [were] triggering cravings. I would get that groggy feeling. I wasn't eating huge amounts, but it doesn't take much to have that sugar hangover. So I decided to give up all processed sugar or alternatives [other than stevia]. I couldn't do it in moderation. And do you know what? I don't miss it."

**My Taste Buds Changed:** "When you're eating sugar, fruit doesn't even register on your palate, because you've numbed your taste buds to anything but the most intense sweet foods. Now, my taste buds have returned to their natural state. Fruit tastes sweet to me. This is not a sacrifice. This is an adventure."

## Initiate The Carb Conversation with Your Family and Friends

If you haven't already done so, you need to talk to family members, roommates, friends, co-workers, or anyone else you deal with regularly. Be ready to explain the new Beyond Sugar Shock journey you're undertaking to improve your health and well-being. In other words, it's time to have what I dub *The Carb Conversation.*

When chatting with those close to you, be honest, loving, composed, and straightforward. Speak from your heart, and let them know how important it is to you—and to them—to be sugar-free or near sugar-free. Most important, tell them you'd really appreciate their loving support and encouragement as you go on your adventure.

Calmly explain that it would be *absolute torture* for you to be surrounded by temptation, because that would be just like offering a recovering alcoholic a glass of wine. Spelling things out clearly in this manner helps your loved ones to understand just how serious you are and how absolutely vital their support is to your success.

But don't be surprised if your friends and family are resistant to helping you give up sweets. Many of them may be hooked themselves. Ultimately, you may need to quit or cut back on sugar *with or without* the support of those around you.

Like a recovering alcoholic or former smoker, you may find it easier to avoid your carb-addicted friends and colleagues until you feel strong enough to handle the temptations.

**YOU'RE A HAPPY, SUCCESSFUL SUGAR KICKER WHEN . . .**
You're okay with the fact that your loved ones don't understand your sugar situation.

That's why, as I stress later in Step 4, it's really important to get consistent support from a therapist, health coach, or life coach; as well as from the Beyond Sugar Shock Freedom community on SparkPeople, the SmartHabitFans on Facebook, or other groups.

Just remember, only others in your predicament can *really* understand your challenges, frustrations, and goals. Now, it's time to prepare for The Carb Conversation with your loved ones.

## Adventurcise: Whom to Approach for The Carb Conversation

With whom would it be useful to disclose your sugar-kicking journey?

1. _____

2. _____

3. _____

4. _____

5. _____

Thoughts/Conclusions

_____

_____

## Adventurcise: What to Say to Loved Ones

Before starting The Carb Conversation, make a list of important points to make when talking with your loved ones.

1. _____

2. _____

3. _____

4. _____

5. _____

Thoughts/Conclusions

_____

_____

# JIMMY MOORE

## SWEET SUCCESS STORY

### "My Wife's Loving Support Helped Me Lose 180 Pounds"

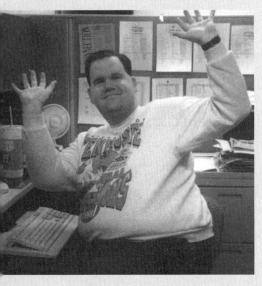

*Note from Connie: In 2004, Jimmy Moore topped the scales at 410 pounds. After a year on the Atkins Diet, he shed 180 pounds and his waist size shrank by 20 inches. He now runs the Livin' La Vida Low Carb blog, at www.livinlavidalowcarb.com. Here's his story.*

**A Pudgy Child Helped Motivate Me:** "I was substitute teaching and writing instructions on the chalkboard when all of a sudden, this pudgy sixth-grade boy exclaimed, 'Mr. Moore is *faaaaat.*' The class burst into laughter, and so did I. But I was only laughing to keep from crying, because that child was right. I was fat, and it was high time I did something about it."

**Sugar Was Killing Me:** "When I started the Atkins Diet on January 1, 2004, one of the first things I did was stop eating sugar. That's when I realized that I had become morbidly obese because of all the sugar I was getting from soft drinks, donuts, cookies, ice cream, and candy bars. And that's why I had high cholesterol, high blood pressure, and difficulty breathing."

**My Wife Was So Supportive:** "My wife, Christine, was worried about my dying early. When I went on the Atkins Diet, she was always there flooding me with encouragement, love, and support. 'You're doing really great!' she'd say. She kept me going and helped strengthen my resolve."

**How My Health Improved:** "The list of benefits goes on and on! I've stabilized my blood sugar, I'm thinking clearer, sex with my wife became more energetic and long lasting, and I have no more aches and pains."

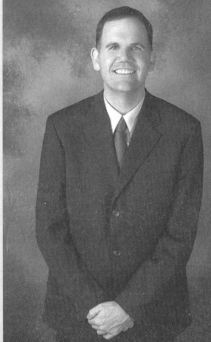

Photos Courtesy of Jimmy Moore

## STEP 4: TEAM UP WITH EXPERTS & SEEK SUPPORT

# Affirmation: I'm easily finding the right people to support me in quitting sugar.

As you begin to sever your overzealous connection to sweets and fast carbs, you can have more far-reaching and lasting success when you get help from understanding professionals such as doctors, health coaches, life coaches, therapists, or nutritionists. In addition, you want to reach out to people who are in your shoes—in other words, fellow Sugar Kickers.

## Work with a Doctor Who Understands Sugar Issues

First and foremost, it's important to find a physician who believes in sugar addiction. Working with a sugar-savvy doctor is critical, as both my coaching clients and I have found.

"A doctor can help you discover the underlying causes for your blood-sugar issues," points out integrative physician Jacob Teitelbaum, M.D., an expert in the relationship between sugar and chronic illness.

Ideally, you want to see a holistic or naturopathic physician, because "they're more likely to be familiar with these conditions," adds Dr. Teitelbaum, a former sugar addict himself and author of *Beat Sugar Addiction Now!*

To get help finding a doctor who "gets it," read the "How to Find a Smart, Sugar-Savvy Doctor" post on my Sugar Shock Blog at www.SugarShockBlog.com.

## Therapy Can Help You Discover Why You "Need" Sugar

If you suspect that you have a sugar addiction or an eating disorder, going into therapy with a trained professional such as a psychologist, psychiatrist, or clinical social worker can help you understand why you turn to your unhealthy carb behavior to cope. A therapist can guide you to face your feelings, deal with grief or self-esteem issues, and look objectively at yourself.

For my part, seeing a therapist or coach was very instrumental in helping me to rise above my sugar dependency for good.

## Consider Hiring a Health Coach

YOU'RE A HAPPY, SUCCESSFUL SUGAR KICKER WHEN ...

You look forward to sharing your successes with your Health Coach, Life Coach, or therapist.

These days, more and more people are relying on health coaches to help them shed excess weight; break their addictions; get more energy; and avoid, reverse, or manage chronic diseases. A health coach—as I discovered while training at the Institute for Integrative Nutrition—can guide and support you while you take small steps in an effective wellness plan so that you don't feel overwhelmed.

Your health coach can help you choose the best tools to let go of your sugar cravings; the ideal techniques to manage your stress; easy, tasty, healthy snacks to bring with you when you're out and about; and the best, most fun activities to nourish you in nonsugary ways so you'll achieve that wonderful Mind-Body-Spirit balance.

What's more, a health coach also can help you phase in other positive, smart habits so you'll make lasting changes that stick.

## Life Coaches Can Move You Forward, Too

Life coaching is another effective process that can help you release your sugar addiction and resolve other issues.

By the way, I'm *both* a certified life coach and a certified health coach so I offer my own special form of Sugar Freedom Coaching and Smart Habits Coaching that is personalized for each client.

To help you learn what life coaching is, let me tell you what it's not. Life coaching is not therapy or counseling, which help you deal with deep, unresolved mental or psychological issues. Often, the focus of therapy or counseling is to help you become much more *functional,* but life coaching—as I learned while studying at the Institute for Professional Excellence in Coaching—helps functional people to live truly *extraordinary* lives.

I recommend both therapy *and* coaching. At times, I may suggest clients also see a therapist, and likewise, therapists may refer coaching clients to me.

Ultimately, we life coaches believe that you, the client, are the expert. You have the inner wisdom and answers to whatever situation you're facing.

It's my role, then, to ask my clients *the right questions* to empower them to access their higher coach. Then together, we'll create your powerful, customized solution.

# DAWN STRICKLAND

### "How Coaching with Connie Helped Me Finally Quit Sugar for Good"

*Note from Connie: When Dawn Strickland (www.GetFitWithDrDawn.com) first came to me for help, she felt completely trapped by her sugar addiction. At publication, Dawn is celebrating more than three years sugar-free.*

**My Sugar Addiction Trapped Me for Years:** "I've struggled with a sugar addiction for as long as I can remember—even though I'm not overweight. During the last ten years, my sugar addiction became much worse. I was always exhausted and hungry, I would cry for no reason, I had horrible PMS every month, and I was easily irritated. I just couldn't handle my demanding life, with two young children, a husband, and a career as a chiropractor and fitness expert. My sugar addiction caused me so much sadness, time, money, and energy."

**My Sugar Binge Drove Me to Find Help:** "One night after a sugar binge, I did a Google search and found Connie's website. Before, I'd only given up sugar for a few weeks or months at a time. This time, I decided that I needed help and had to *commit* to quit *for good.*"

**My Husband & Friends Didn't Understand My Sugar Addiction:** "They'd say, 'Just eat a little dessert,' but I couldn't. They didn't realize that I was just like an alcoholic but with sugar. I needed to be accountable to someone who really understood it, especially on days when I was at my lowest, and that someone was Connie."

**Knowing What to Do Wasn't Enough:** "Just reading Connie's book *Sugar Shock!* wasn't enough for me. I needed personal help to get out of my vicious cycle. While it hasn't always been easy, I couldn't have kicked sugar without Connie's coaching. She supported me through tough times and helped me create a personalized plan that worked for me."

## Nutritionists Can Help You, Too

After my doctor ordered me to quit sugar in 1998, one of the first things I did was see a nutritionist. She helped me figure out how much protein to eat, how often to snack, how to choose well-balanced meals and snacks, and what to do if I felt weak.

You also may wish to see a certified nutrition consultant, who can suggest, along with your doctor, what tests to take to find allergies or sensitivities, and which supplements or herbs might be ideal for you.

### COACH CONNIE'S SWEET SUCCESS STRATEGY

### Buddy Up Both Online & In Person for More Support

While you sever your attachment to sweets and quickie carbs, the best way to stay upbeat, motivated, and on track is to buddy up with other people who are equally determined to shed their sugar habit or excess weight.

It's much easier to dissolve your habit if you can call or e-mail a Break-Free Buddy when sweets beckon. And, if you live in the same area, you can even meet a buddy at the gym, a hiking trail, or a park for a workout.

You want a number of positive-thinking people, who can support and encourage you when you're in need. Ideally you should try to find others also doing this Beyond Sugar Shock program, because they can remind you about cool tools to use and share firsthand experiences. Likewise, you'll be there for them when they want your help, too.

It's also a good idea to connect with successful people who've already gone sugar-free. Naturally, when you're facing challenging situations, your Break-Free Buddies will be there for you, too.

Research supports the importance of such buddies. For instance, a study in the *Archives of Internal Medicine* showed that teaming up with others—either family or friends—can result in greater weight loss when their partners are also gung ho and successful themselves.

## Get Sparked to Reach Your Goals on SparkPeople.com

Thanks to the Internet, you can easily connect with like-minded people confronting the same issues. SparkPeople, America's largest free diet and fitness website, offers a way to interact with millions of people worldwide—from the comfort of your own home.

A study for the *International Journal of Medical Informatics* showed that the site—which primarily draws women—played a prominent role in helping participants achieve their goals. More than 87 percent of those surveyed appreciated the encouragement and motivation on the forums, 58.5 percent loved the information, and 42.5 percent valued the shared experiences.

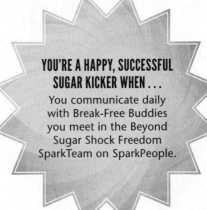

**YOU'RE A HAPPY, SUCCESSFUL SUGAR KICKER WHEN . . .**
You communicate daily with Break-Free Buddies you meet in the Beyond Sugar Shock Freedom SparkTeam on SparkPeople.

"We're sparking people to reach their goals," explains "SparkGuy" Chris Downie, the site's founder, CEO, and a motivational expert, speaking on my *Gab with the Gurus Radio Show*.

"We focus on what you *can* do," says Downie, author of *The New York Times* best-selling book, *The Spark*. "We encourage people to take small steps and then build on that momentum. Those small sparks eventually lead to major breakthroughs."

---

## Get Support from the Beyond Sugar Shock Freedom SparkTeam on SparkPeople

I'm deeply committed to offering free online support to those of you in need. In 2002, I founded my first group, KickSugar on Yahoo, to help people like you as much as possible. The group—which has since moved to SparkPeople.com—offers you a chance to participate in challenges with other people, who also seek to move beyond sugar.

In the Beyond Sugar Shock Freedom SparkTeam, you can get or give nurturing and encouragement at any time of day or night; discover easy, healthy snack foods and SWEET meals; post your favorite sugar-free recipes and find new dishes to try; and much more.

Of course, my Beyond Sugar Shock Freedom SparkTeam team and I also share valuable, easy-to-do, quit-sugar tips with you, too. You can also use SparkPeople's other features, such as the popular Nutrition Tracker to monitor your food and water intake and read informative articles from health experts.

I invite you: Join us, the Beyond Sugar Shock Freedom SparkTeam, now. To be a part of our community, just visit http://teams.sparkpeople.com/BeyondSugarShock.

By the way, we're always seeking Community Leaders, so you can help yourself and others at the same time. To get involved with the Beyond Sugar Shock Freedom SparkTeam, just post something on my Facebook fan page (SmartHabitsFans).

Speaking of Facebook, you're also invited to chat with us often there. I'm quite active on the SmarHabitsFans Facebook page. Visit me there, and get links to Woo-Hoo, Feel-Good Tunes; daily motivational thoughts; cool videos; provocative questions that invite you to reply; a chance to post your gratitude musings; and much more.

# TIFFANY MONIQUE

### A Backup Singer for Beyoncé Sheds Weight with Support at SparkPeople

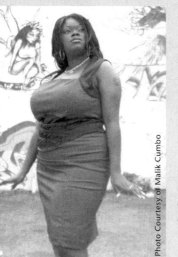

Photo Courtesy of Malik Cumbo

*Note from Connie: When singer/songwriter Tiffany Monique (www. tiffanymonique.com) joined Beyoncé's background vocalist trio, The Mamas, her career began to take off. Says Beyoncé: "Tiffany's voice has effortless strength, sass, seduction, and heart with a tone that puts you at ease." But at 235 pounds, the 5'3" singer—who'd been diagnosed as prediabetic—was worried about not having the range, stamina, and confidence she needed; not being able to keep up with her young son; and getting type 2 diabetes, which had killed her grandparents. As she revealed on my Gab with the Gurus Radio Show, Tiffany found a nurturing community on www.Sparkpeople.com.*

**My Nemesis Was Sugar:** "Sugar was absolutely the number one problem I had. It took learning more about its effects on my body and accepting the fact that I ate entirely too much candy, cookies, and especially ice cream [before I could quit it]. I absolutely, positively do not eat junk food and ice cream anymore. I can't have it, because I will abuse it. Not even a little, not even as a treat."

**Beyoncé Is Committed to Health:** "Before I was following my weight-loss path, most of us would have pizza and French fries [while on the road], but Beyoncé always ate salads and other healthy foods and didn't even seem tempted. She was that focused and committed to her health and fitness."

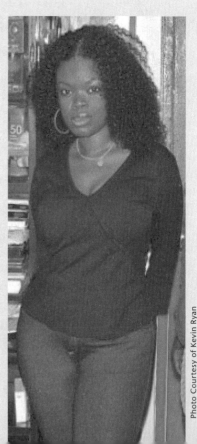

Photo Courtesy of Kevin Ryan

**I'm Healthy Now:** "I now have a clean bill of health. The prediabetes diagnosis went away, and my cholesterol and blood pressure have gone down. Plus, the numbness in my limbs and the rheumatoid arthritis in my knee have disappeared. And I can now move around the stage, dance, and not be winded."

**Why I Love SparkPeople:** "One thing that appeals to me is that www.SparkPeople.com is free. Money I'd normally have to spend on membership costs I can now use to buy healthier foods. I also like the encouragement and accountability that it promotes with its fun SparkPoint system in which you're rewarded often."

**My SparkBuddies Cheer Me On:** "Now, as people learn more about my personal journey, they will not let me slip. An hour doesn't go by that I don't hear from someone on SparkPeople saying, 'Wow, you look great! Keep going!' Or 'I've been trying to lose weight for years and now that I read your story, I think that I can do it, too.' People genuinely want to see you succeed. So I'm a SparkPerson for life."

This week, you made some important, but subtle changes to bolster your mind-set and attitude. I invite you to answer these questions. If you forgot to do any of these fun things, just go back and do them now. As you read through these questions, feel free to jot notes to yourself either in this book or in your journal.

## Before You Head into Week Two, Have you Laid the Groundwork for Your Success?

- Are you boogying to your Woo-Hoo, Feel-Good Theme Song every day and doing the Success Strut?

- Do you boldly pronounce your affirmations frequently throughout your day?

- Do you regularly See, Feel & Act As If You've Already Won?

- Are you looking at your vision board several minutes a day?

- Are you regularly doing Sugary Soul Searching?

- Are you often asking yourself the 5 W's & 1 H?

- Did you prepare your "Why I Need to Quit" and Benefits lists, and are you taking it with you for inspiration wherever you go?

- Have you made an appointment with a sugar-savvy doctor yet?

- Have you found a supportive therapist, health coach, life coach, or nutritionist?

- Have you joined the free Beyond Sugar Shock Freedom SparkTeam on www.SparkPeople.com and started chatting with us?

## Congratulations! You've Completed Week One

Pat yourself on the back. You've made an important commitment to your health and happiness by making it through the first week of your Beyond Sugar Shock program. Now, it's time to put your positive energy and focus on your beautiful body.

## CHAPTER 6

## WEEK TWO

# YOUR BODY: CHOOSE SMARTER HABITS & BEGIN BETTER FOOD BEHAVIOR

**Affirmation: I'm now choosing smarter, healthier habits to release Sugar Shock.**

As you enter the second week of our adventure together, you'll start focusing on your body. It's important to honor this marvelous temple of yours, which has worked so hard for you all these years despite all your poor food decisions.

This week, you'll also decide how you'll quit sugar and quickie carbs. Will you simply go cold turkey or opt for a more gradual approach?

Remember: letting go of your sugar habit isn't so much about *moving away* from fast, fiber-poor, nutrient-deprived foods as it is about *moving toward* foods and activities that can bring you good health and sweetness.

You want to begin taking a more deliberate, joyous approach toward food, which you'll now choose more carefully. A simple rule of thumb for eating better foods is to fill your plate at each meal with ample tasty produce, quality sources of protein, and modest amounts of healthy fats.

While you're transitioning from S.A.D. to SWEET foods during these first three weeks of the program, you can even "sin" and "cheat" on purpose, if you so choose.

You read right! I'll show you how to indulge—politely—in sugar and carbs from time to time during this period. However, if you're a Red-Lighter around sweets, you may not want to risk it.

As you begin to replace high-sugar, high-salt, processed nonfoods with more robust, flavorful, satisfying alive foods—and completely switch over by Week Four—you'll feel more energized and satisfied after you eat. Very soon, you'll notice that as your taste buds change, you simply won't crave those S.A.D. foods anymore.

Now here are your four steps for Week Two.

Week Two: **YOUR BODY**
**STEP 1:** Start a Love Affair—with Your Body
**STEP 2:** Personalize Your Program—Decide How You'll Quit
**STEP 3:** Write Off Your Sugar Habit & Your Weight—and Shed Twice as Much!
**STEP 4:** Do Polite "Sugar Sinning" & Other Smart Moves

## STEP 1: START A LOVE AFFAIR—WITH YOUR BODY

### Affirmation: I love and approve of my body— especially my stomach, butt, and hips.

It's time to shift from using or abusing sweets and quickie carbs to honoring and appreciating your body and the real you. This week, you want to fall head over heels in love with yourself. As you go about your day—while you take a bath, do laundry, go for a walk, or pass a mirror—you'll only think and say positive, loving things about yourself.

Do you find it challenging to imagine saying lovey-dovey things to yourself? Then just pretend that you're your own amazing lover, who makes you sigh, smile, or moan contentedly.

To kick sugar or shed weight, it's absolutely *vital* that you practice self-love and appreciate your body as it is. In other words, become your Constant Sweetie. Remind yourself often just how great you are. For instance, say, *[Your Name], you're so fun, sexy, and slim.* Choose phrases that appeal to you.

**YOU'RE A HAPPY, SUCCESSFUL SUGAR KICKER WHEN . . .**
You love, appreciate, and praise your body daily.

## Affirmation: I bless my body with love and kindness.

### Mirror Love Affirmations

Part of learning to adore yourself is to do frequent Mirror Love Affirmations, something Louise Hay suggests. Every time you pass a mirror, look deep into your eyes and lavish kind words on various parts of your body, especially those areas you feel insecure about or downright hate.

Tell yourself you have *nice arms, hot legs,* or *a great butt.* In some cases, you may be projecting yourself into the future (because you're not there yet). In other instances, pay attention to the body part you do like but usually don't appreciate, like your eyes, your lips, or your hair.

While you gaze adoringly at yourself in the mirror, extend your love to your whole being. Heaping appreciative attention on your body is an important part of being able to release your sugar addiction.

And if you want to shed flab and fat, expressing body love can put you in the right frame of mind to succeed.

### Playcise: Become Your Constant Sweetie: How Do I Love Thee?

What do you most love about your body?

1._____

2._____

3._____

What do you most love about your personality?

1._____

2._____

3._____

What will you do to shower yourself in love?

1._____

2._____

3 _____

Now, you'll conclude Step 1 in Week Two with another fun Adventurcise. You'll write your body a love letter.

## Adventurcise: Love Away Your Fat & Sugar Habit: Write Your Body a Love Letter

It's time to graciously give your body a very special gift. You'll write it a love letter, in which you apologize and pledge to cherish, revere, and bless it, as well as give it the gratitude, adoration, and devotion it deserves.

Just use the love letter on the next page and add your own promises. Or create your own, but make sure to address three topics in it.

First, thank your body for always being there for you. Second, sincerely apologize to your poor body for having abused it so often. And third, promise to treat it much better and to do your best to bring about radiant health.

Put your Dearest Body Letter (which, by the way, is an idea inspired by the Institute for Integrative Nutrition) in a safe, private place such as your nightstand. Your love letter will gently remind you to be consciously sweet to your body on a consistent basis.

Dearest Wonderful Body of Mine,

I love you so much. I'm so awed and amazed at how loyally you've served me all these years. I wouldn't be here if it weren't for you.

Because of you, I can breathe, move, and turn foods I eat into energy, excitement, and joy.

Dearest Body, I want to apologize from the bottom of my heart for taking you for granted and for consistently abusing you by filling you with so much sugar and so many candies, culprit carbs, and other S.A.D. nonfoods. [Add other things you may have done to harm your body—for instance, if you've smoked cigarettes, or drunk too much alcohol or caffeine, mention that, too.]

Please, forgive me, Dearest Body.

I'm now determined to change things. I hereby promise and pledge to:

- Thank you every day with heartfelt gratitude that you're here for me.

- Love, honor, respect, cherish, and appreciate you for all you do.

- Face up to the fact that for years, I've mindlessly pumped you full of dangerous, life-shortening foods.

- Fully forgive myself for treating you like a trash can or rotting garbage heap.

- Do *all* I can to heal you and make you healthy, such as see a doctor, take supplements, create a vision board, and complete this Beyond Sugar Shock program.

- Tap into my inner strength so that I can overcome this sugar and carb addiction that hurts you so much.

- Find sweet, nurturing, non-food-related ways to give you the laughter, fun, play, and pleasure that make you feel good.

- Exercise regularly and appropriately for my body type.

- Give you all the sleep you need every night and the relaxation you require in between.

- Be grateful for you just the way you are.

- Tune in daily to get messages you send to me when you're hurt or sick so I can discover what you really need and want.

- Understand that my unexpressed or ignored emotions and thoughts hurt you.

Add additional promises, if you like.

- _____

- _____


Dearest Body, I love you so much,

Your Name  _____

Date  _____

## STEP 2: PERSONALIZE YOUR PROGRAM— DECIDE HOW YOU'LL QUIT

## Affirmation: I'm finding the perfect kick-sugar plan for me.

For many, taking sweets out of your life is comparable to quitting cigarettes, coffee, or alcohol. Some people prefer to do it all at once and just get it over with quickly, while others like to wean themselves off slowly.

It's now time to create your personalized Break-Free Plan. You can tackle this in one of three ways.

1. Quit sugar cold turkey.

2. Kick gradually, slowly phasing sugar out of your life.

3. Drastically curtail your intake of sweets, but still permit yourself occasional tastes.

Over the years, I've talked with fans of all three approaches. Anita Flegg, 43, decided to quit all at once. "I'd tried cold turkey many times before, but this time I was very careful to eat a protein snack every two hours to help keep up my blood-sugar levels," recalls Anita, author of *Hypoglycemia: The Other Sugar Disease*.

"The most important thing, though, was how I 'sold' it to myself. I kept saying *I won't eat sugar today. Tomorrow, who knows! But for today, I won't have any.* I still talk to myself that way."

Ruth M., 53, chose the phase-out approach. "I once thought I couldn't go through life without my sugar fix, but by taking sugar out gradually, cushioning the shock of withdrawal with fruit and, of course, eating proper protein meals, I got there. Life is so very, very much better now."

By the way, even top medical experts are divided on the most effective way to quit The Sweet Stuff. For example, Fred Pescatore, M.D., former associate medical director of the Atkins Center and author of *The Hamptons Diet*, maintains that "quitting cold turkey is the best way because after three days the craving is gone. The drawback to cutting down gradually is that it takes so long, and the dependence doesn't go away as quickly."

Among those who advocate going slowly is one of my mentors, Nancy Appleton, Ph.D., author of *Suicide by Sugar*. "When you go cold turkey, you start secreting the wrong amount of hormones due to all the sugar you've been consuming. This causes withdrawal symptoms," she explains.

And, at this point, she says, people might fail. "They get scared because they experience withdrawal symptoms like headaches, fatigue, perspiration, and anger. So they may go back to eating sugar again," Dr. Appleton warns. "But if you cut it out slowly, your pancreas, thyroid, pituitary, and adrenal glands have time to readjust."

The concept of permitting yourself periodic desserts also has its share of medical supporters, including cardiologist and antiaging specialist Stephen Sinatra, M.D., the medical consultant for my first book, *Sugar Shock!*

Dr. Sinatra thinks it's more realistic to follow an 80/20 rule, which means you'll eat healthily 80 percent of the time and allow yourself occasional indulgences the other 20 percent. Your periodic "cheats" make it easier to eat well the rest of the time, he contends.

Still, for many, "planned indulging" is like opening Pandora's Box, as clients have often shared with me. It's sort of like a recovering alcoholic who decides, *Ah heck, I'll treat myself with just one drink*. And, of course, we know that this almost always triggers a full-scale binge.

If you're a Red-Lighter around sweets and one bite always leads to more, then you may need to quit sugar cold turkey. Trying to taper off or have periodic indulgences can be too risky, especially if you've been battling your sugar habit for years.

Also, I strongly advise you to go cold turkey as soon as possible if you have pressing medical reasons to avoid sweets, such as a metabolic disorder, type 2 diabetes, hypoglycemia, or heart disease.

Of course, if you're a Green-Lighter or Yellow-Lighter, you can quit sugar all at once, taper off gradually, or even allow yourself tastes a few times a year.

In fact, for some, occasional, deliberate "cheating"—polite portions please!—may ensure that you stay sugar-free most of the time.

## Consider Your Commitments & Lifestyle

To be successful, you'll want to follow a kick-sugar approach that best suits your personality, work schedule, family obligations, and other commitments. Quitting cold turkey may be ideal for you if you have a flexible schedule, can rearrange your duties and obligations, can take a vacation day or two from work, and have sup-portive family members willing to take up some of the slack.

On the other hand, if you have a rigorous schedule—a demanding job; kids to carpool to school, soccer, or dance lessons; meals to prepare for the family; or other can't-miss commitments—you may find it more workable to stop gradually.

For instance, you can begin by limiting yourself to one or two sugary foods or quickie carbs per day, having maybe six bites. Then you can slowly taper off to, at most, four bites of one type of dessert food or several sips of a sugary beverage. Next, you can keep scaling back until you're not consuming any sugar or quickie carbs at all.

Whichever method you choose, keep in mind that it may take some trial and error before you determine what's right for you.

And remember: however you decide to quit, you won't actually do so until Week Four of the program. Right now, your job is to explore options, figure out what makes sense for you, and set a path that will ensure your success.

Now, let's consider the pros and cons of the various methods of removing sugar from your life.

| Kicking Sugar Cold Turkey: Pros and Cons | |
|---|---|
| **Pros:** | **Cons:** |
| • You'll quickly detox your body and get it back on track. Once you get through the discomfort of withdrawal, life will get great *fast!* | • Withdrawal symptoms—headaches, exhaustion, irritability, difficulty con-centrating, and cravings—could be intense. (Soon I'll give you many sugar-kicking tips to help diminish these symptoms.) |
| • You don't have to worry about what to do around sweets—you just know that you won't have any. | • During your first few days off sugar, you may feel strong cravings to eat something sugary just to relieve your withdrawal symptoms, but remember, relying on sweets won't help in the long run. In fact, if you do eat dessert foods, your symptoms will quickly re-turn, perhaps even worse than before. |
| • Quitting cold turkey allows your taste buds to change more quickly so that you don't crave sweet foods the way you once did. | • Stress might be tough to handle while you're quitting, so you'll need to learn better ways to cope. (You'll soon get helpful tools to relax and manage your sugar tension.) |

## Kicking Sugar Gradually: Pros and Cons

| Pros: | Cons: |
|---|---|
| • Cutting back slowly gives your poor, abused body a chance to adjust, which means you'll have far fewer, if any, withdrawal symptoms so you'll function better while you're kicking. | • You'll continue to expose your body to Sugar Shock, and it will take much longer to get sugar totally out of your life. |
| • Going slowly gives you a chance to gradually change your eating habits, build mental fortitude, and not feel "deprived." | • You may remain tempted by the allure of sugar. Some folks find that one bite always leads to more, so it's hard for them to just cut back. The sweet taste of dessert foods could trigger more sugar cravings. |
| • Kicking sugar gradually allows you to surround yourself with loved ones and Break-Free Buddies who can support you in your endeavor. | • Your taste buds won't change as quickly as they would if you quit cold turkey. |

## Taking Sweet Tastes Now and Then: Pros and Cons

| Pros: | Cons: |
|---|---|
| • You'll never feel deprived because you know that up to about six times a year, you can take up to four small bites of dessert. | • You may not be able to stop at just four bites. It can be downright frustrating— if not maddening and disheartening— to have only a few tastes. |
| • You can feel at home at a business function, celebration, or party when everyone else around you is eating sweets. | • You may be left with a feeling of *always wanting more*, which may trigger a pity party. And, of course, we don't want that! |
| • You won't dread the idea of never being able to indulge again. | • You may spend too much time plotting your next sugar tasting, which means you're still placing way too much emphasis and emotional charge into your sugar habit. |

Now it's time for you decide how to quit. What method is best for you?

## Adventurcise: Weigh Your Pros and Cons

You've already determined if you're a Green-, Yellow-, or Red-Lighter when it comes to sweets and quickie carbs. Now, with that in mind, weigh the pros and cons of each method. Whatever approach you opt to take, please see your doctor first to discuss your decision.

Quit Cold Turkey _____ Phase It Out Gradually _____

Taste Sweets Now and Then_____

Why?

1._____

2._____

3._____

Now look at a calendar to find the actual date when you'll start Week Four of the Beyond Sugar Shock program (roughly two weeks from today).

That's the day you'll Break Free!

It's time to make a photocopy of this pledge and sign it. You may wish to share it with a buddy or loved one, too.

## My Sugar-Free Success Pledge

I, _____ (name), hereby decide to make drastic changes in my sugar consumption. I intend to become sweetly sugar-free or mostly sugar-free.

I Will Quit Cold Turkey _____ Cut Back Gradually _____

Have Occasional Tastes _____

I Will Start on This Date: _____, 20_____

(My name)_____

(My signature) _____

(Date) _____ , 20_____

(Witnessed by/optional)_____

## STEP 3: WRITE OFF YOUR SUGAR HABIT & YOUR WEIGHT—AND SHED TWICE AS MUCH!

### Affirmation: I joyously write down everything I eat and drink.

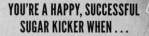

**YOU'RE A HAPPY, SUCCESSFUL SUGAR KICKER WHEN . . .**

You make a plan and set a date to remove sugar from your life.

When it comes to weight loss, the pen is mightier than the scale. Now, you want to begin to keep careful track of *everything* you put into your mouth, including beverages. Being accountable to yourself in this way will be an eye-opening experience, because it will force you to come face-to-face with your total consumption, especially those mindless late-afternoon or late-evening snacks you shove down while on autopilot.

In fact, every day, you make more than 200 choices about what to eat, but you're aware of only a fraction of these food decisions, according to food psychologist Brian Wansink, Ph.D., director of the Cornell University Food and Brand Lab, and author of *Mindless Eating: Why We Eat More Than We Think.*

Consider a few mindless decisions you may have made this week: You *decided* to buy that bag of chocolate-covered peanuts from the work vending machine after a nerve-wracking conversation with your boss. You *decided* to eat potato chips before dinner. You *decided* to eat the entire portion of white-flour pasta over Sunday lunch with your family.

Keeping a food journal is a surefire way to become a Conscious Quality Eater.

Not only that, but a study from Kaiser Permanente Center for Health Research of nearly 1,700 overweight and obese adults, revealed those who kept daily food records *lost twice as much weight* as those who kept no records. The people who kept track six or more days per week lost 18 pounds over a six-month period while nontrackers shed only 9 pounds.

Convinced yet about the value of keeping track?

# ANN COOK

## A Food Diary Helped Me Lose Nearly 150 Pounds

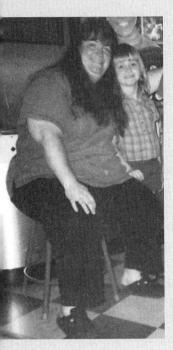

**My Rock Bottom Moment:** "In spring 2008, I literally lay dying in a tiny cape house in Sebago, Maine. I weighed about 300 pounds, had severe type 2 diabetes (which required up to 15 doses of three different types of insulin per day), severe asthma (for which I needed two different inhalers), and debilitating depression. Plus, I was trapped in a very abusive marriage and had six children, then aged 4 to 11."

*Extreme Makeover: Home Edition* **Woke Me Up:** "When my children and I were on vacation in Maynard, Massachusetts, we learned that *Extreme Makeover: Home Edition* was filming. We volunteered every day to help build the house. This gave me something else to think about rather than food."

**My Desire to Be Healthier Motivated Me:** "To lose weight, I kept a laserlike focus. Nothing else mattered. I wanted the end result—a healthy, desirable body—more than I've ever wanted anything before."

**150 Pounds Came Right Off:** "I lost weight *The Biggest Loser*-style without ever being on the TV show. I eliminated refined carbohydrates and foods with added sugars; restricted calories; ate real, whole foods; and began exercising—a lot. I lost almost 150 pounds and shrank from a size 28 to a size 2. I've now maintained my weight loss for three years and haven't had a single donut, drop of soda, or bite of fast food."

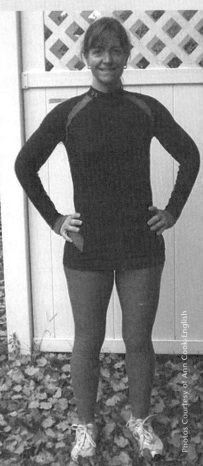

**Keeping a Food Diary Made the Difference:** "During my entire journey, I kept a small notebook with me at all times and wrote down *everything* I ate and drank. I also tracked my exercise, thoughts, emotions, and weight. Journaling helped keep me accountable, provided valuable information, and offered me a place to vent both positive and negative emotions. I also started a blog (http://imaphoenixbaby.blogspot.com/) to share my journey with others."

**My Health Turned Around:** "I've gone from nearly dying to being vibrantly healthy. I no longer have asthma and show no signs of ever having been diabetic. I continue to eat well and exercise daily. I'm an avid runner, and I enjoy cycling, strength training, hiking, long walks, kayaking, and camping."

**Kicking Sweets Changed Me in Other Ways, Too:** "Not only did I break free of my sugar and carb habit, but I ended my abusive marriage and returned to school. I hope to study medicine, because I want to help prevent and cure obesity."

Photos Courtesy of Ann Cook-English

## How Your Food Journal Will Help You Quit Sugar

If you religiously write down everything you eat or drink, your food journal helps you become more mindful. For instance, it helps you to pinpoint where you're getting those "little" extras—say, the four teaspoons of sugar that you slipped into your French vanilla, whipped cream–topped coffee drink.

You'll also discover what times of day or night are trickiest for you and when you're most at risk of overeating. Or maybe you'll learn you're an emotional eater, who turns to food even if you're not hungry. If you're headed toward a binge, writing down what you *want* to eat can help "wake you up" first.

In addition, keeping a food journal can remind you to round out meals with adequate protein, fat, quality carbs, and fiber, and to pick appropriate portion sizes. You can also track your aerobic exercise and weight training.

> **YOU'RE A HAPPY, SUCCESSFUL SUGAR KICKER WHEN . . .**
>
> It's second nature for you to write down every morsel you eat or sip you take.

## Start to Keep Track at Your Next Meal or Snack

It's now time to start keeping track, but first, you need to decide how to do it. For example, you can fill out separate Beyond Sugar Shock Food-to-Mood Tracker sheets. (Just photocopy the one provided on the next page.) Or you could jot down your food intake in your phone or calendar. Just keep track in whatever way works best for you. Now, for a few simple guidelines:

- *Record* every single time you put something into your mouth—foods or beverages.

- *Answer the 5 W's & 1 H.* Jot down *who* you're with, *what* you're doing, and *what* is eating you, if anything; *when* you're eating; *where* you are; *why* you're eating and *why* now; and *how* you feel beforehand and afterward.

- *Evaluate, then Reevaluate.* After a few days of keeping track, review your entries to identify patterns. Are you skipping breakfast and lunch, and then overeating at dinner? Do you grab a sugary snack at 2 P.M. or 10 P.M.? Do certain people set you off? Do you start eating when you're tired, upset, or nervous? Once you discover your weak points, find better options such as taking a nap if you're tired, calling a friend if you're lonely, or crying if you're sad.

Below you'll find the Beyond Sugar Shock Food-to-Mood Tracker, which will help you gain wonderful insights about how you *use* sweets and carbs. After just a couple of days or a week or two of tracking, you'll know much more about yourself and what triggers your eating habits, and you'll no longer need to keep as detailed a record. However, you'll still want to track all foods and beverages you consume.

## The Beyond Sugar Shock Food-to-Mood Tracker

Date _____, 20_____

| Time | What I ate (any sugar?), and how I felt physically & emotionally. |
|------|------------------------------------------------------------------|
| 6 A.M. | |
| 7 A.M. | |
| 8 A.M. | |
| 9 A.M. | |
| 10 A.M. | |
| 11 A.M. | |
| 12 noon | |
| 1 P.M. | |
| 2 P.M. | |
| 3 P.M. | |
| 4 P.M. | |
| 5 P.M. | |
| 6 P.M. | |
| 7 P.M. | |
| 8 P.M. | |
| 9 P.M. | |
| 10 P.M. | |
| 11 P.M. | |
| 12 A.M. | |
| 1 A.M. | |
| 2 A.M. | |
| 3 A.M. | |
| 4 A.M. | |
| 5 A.M. | |

My Thoughts & Feelings Today and How My Foods/Drinks Affected Them:

When did I feel best today? Why?

_____

When did I feel worst today? Why?

_____

What were my physical symptoms?

_____

What were my emotional symptoms?

_____

How did I get along with my loved ones and co-workers today?

_____

Did I embarrass myself today or behave in a way unlike me? Was I moody, crabby, angry, irrational, short-fused, confused, or more? Specify.

_____

Did I act this way after having sweets?_____

If so, how much later was it? _____

Was I a zombie at any time today? What did I do to pep myself up?

_____

How many times did I have sugar or refined carbs today? _____

When?_____

How did I feel immediately afterward?_____

How did I feel two hours later?_____

Four hours?_____

Eight hours?_____

What healthy foods did I eat today? _____

_____

How much water did I have today?_____

Were there any trigger situations in which I found myself? What were they?

_____

_____

Did anyone seek to sabotage my efforts (whether consciously or not)? Who?

_____

How can I avoid these situations or people in the future?
_____

Did I feel deprived today? How?
_____

What food(s) agreed with me most?
_____
_____

What food(s) disagreed with me?
_____
_____

What can I do differently tomorrow?
_____
_____

Did I seek support today from others?
_____

How did I treat myself today in nonsugar ways?
_____
_____

Today's most important lesson(s):
_____
_____

What did I do today for which I can pat myself on the back?
_____

What can I do to get support tomorrow?
_____

How can I treat myself tomorrow in sweet, non-food-related ways?
_____
_____
_____
_____
_____
_____

## High-Tech? Keep Track with Web Tools

If you'd rather take a more high-tech approach to keeping track of your intake, you can store your food journal online. Here are some options:

- **SparkPeople** (http://sparkpeople.com/): You can be one of millions to use this site's popular Nutrition Trackers tool. A free mobile app is available. (While there, make sure to join our Beyond Sugar Shock Freedom SparkTeam.)

- **LoseIt** (http://loseit.com/): A popular free mobile app helps you record food and exercise.

- **Daily Burn** (http://dailyburn.com/): A free online program helps you reach your fitness goals, whether you want to build upper body strength or run your first 5k.

- **LiveStrong** (http://www.livestrong.com/thedailyplate/): You can find 1,500 fitness activities in addition to an extensive calorie database.

## STEP 4: Do Polite "Sugar Sinning" & Other Smart Moves

### Affirmation: I am in control. I choose to say no to sweets.

As you begin to choose tasty, nutritious, real foods during these initial three weeks, you may find yourself naturally eating less sugar and fewer carbs. But if you feel tempted and want to "cheat," you need to follow seven simple guidelines.

*Guideline #1: Always eat healthy food first.* Before you even *think* about having any dessert, make sure you've had a well-balanced lunch or dinner—with quality protein, fiber-filled carbs, and healthy fats. These foods won't put you into a yo-yo blood-sugar situation, which could trigger sugar cravings.

*Guideline #2: Partake of polite portions.* Take only up to five small bites twice a day. The following week, scale back to four bites; a week later, to three, etc.

*Guideline #3: Set a curfew and snack smart.* Only have sugary snacks twice a day—after a healthy lunch or dinner. Do *not* allow yourself to eat after 8 or 9 P.M.

*Guideline #4: Slow down and chew with purpose.* While tasting sweets, be mindful, deliberate, and focused. Chew each bite as many times as you can—preferably about 20 to 30 times. Do not watch TV, read, or listen to the radio while noshing. (Shortly, you'll get an easy lesson on how to eat mindfully.)

*Guideline #5: Do Sugary Soul Searching about Your Sugar Sinning.* As soon as you can after a few bites, take out your food journal and write down what you ate, what emotions were triggered, if you felt deprived at having to stop after a few bites, and what you may have learned.

*Guideline #6: Regard sweet tastes as a tool to teach, not reward, yourself.* Viewing sweets as "treats" doled out for good behavior can be counterproductive to your kick-sugar or weight-loss goals. Instead, regard your deliberate Sugar Sinning experiences as lessons, which will give you valuable information so that it'll be easier for you to let go of sweets later.

*Guideline #7: Wisely choose your place to taste and your companion.* Make sure to taste sweets only in a public place such as a restaurant or at a friend's or family member's home. This means absolutely *no eating sweets while alone* or at a crowded party. And do not take leftovers home—that's simply far too tempting and too dangerous!

## As You Begin to Break Up with Sugar, What Sweets Can You Taste?

Now that you understand your Sugar Sinning guidelines, it's a good idea to begin to make healthier, sweet substitutions twice a day. Here are some better choices for dessert, according to Jill Lane, C.N.C., this book's meal consultant.

- 2 ounces of dark chocolate (the less sugar, the better). Go for 65% or higher cocoa content.

- A bowl of berries covered with homemade whipped cream (using only ¼ to ½ teaspoon of sugar, and only if you have no dairy issues).

- A frozen banana with 1 ounce of dark chocolate.

- ¼ cup of dark chocolate–covered nuts.

- Frozen berries with ⅓ cup of plain yogurt (if you can handle dairy) or coconut yogurt.

- Or pick four to five bites twice a day of a dessert of your own choosing.

## Curb the Blood Sugar Bouncers

At this point, you also want to cut back on caffeine and alcohol and, of course, nicotine, which can wreak havoc with your blood-sugar levels. Please note, though, that I'm not suggesting that you totally quit them right away—you have enough on your plate right now—but it's wise to dramatically dial down your blood-sugar-bouncing habits.

Both caffeine and alcohol stimulate cortisol, which makes you secrete too much insulin. That, in turn, can lead to low blood sugar or hypoglycemia symptoms, which means you'll have such ailments as headaches, mood swings, and dizziness. And ultimately these drinks may lead to sugar cravings and bingeing.

## How to Sweeten Beverages During This Phase-Out Period

At this early stage, you also may use some short-term sweetening substitutes to add to your herbal tea or coffee up to twice a day. You can use ¼ to ½ teaspoon of the following:

- Maple syrup

- Organic honey (preferably locally produced and direct from the farmer. Bear in mind that honey is more concentrated than table sugar.)

- Date sugar

- Brown rice syrup

- Sorghum

- Brown cane sugar

- Stevia (You need only a pinch of the noncaloric *Stevia rebaudiana* to sweeten drinks and foods, because in its natural form, it's about 19 times sweeter than sugar. Let a leaf steep in your tea for a minute or two or use ⅛ or ¹⁄₁₆ of a teaspoon [or even less] of the green ground powder. Please note that I suggest using stevia only as it comes from Mother Nature—*in its original green leaf or green powder form.*)

By now, I hope you realize that the purpose of tasting sweets during the first half of this program is to help you *gain control* over your habit and realize that *you can stop.*

Although I'm giving you permission to do polite, selective Sugar Sinning, you simply may not feel comfortable or confident in doing so. That's fine, too. Just continue to enjoy and explore the many other healthy and delicious options available to you.

Now, it's time to decide if you can politely indulge.

## Adventurcise: Can You Do Polite Sugar Sinning?

Yes, I can do it. Here's why:

_____

_____

No, I can't do it! Here's why:

_____

_____

## COACH CONNIE'S SWEET SUCCESS STRATEGY

### Become a Smart Sugar Sleuth

Now that you're on your way to ditching or phasing out sugar, you need to become what I call a *Smart Sugar Sleuth* so that you know how to read and interpret food labels.

For instance, be on the lookout for sugars that are added to allegedly healthy energy bars, yogurts, and whole-grain breakfast cereals.

To begin, you want to know that:

- All food labels list sugar content in grams, not ounces. To get a close approximation of how many teaspoons that is, just divide the number of grams in sugar by four. (One teaspoon equals roughly four grams.)

- As of this writing, there's no distinction on U.S. food labels between added sugars and naturally occurring sugars. (The CSPI vainly petitioned the FDA in 1999 to require that labels specify how much sugar has been added to foods and drinks.)

## COACH CONNIE'S SWEET SUCCESS STRATEGY

- Hidden sugars are added to thousands of salad dressings, yogurts, frozen foods, breads, soups, sauces, and fast foods such as French fries and hot dogs. Just assume that when it comes to processed foods, nine times out of ten, some type of sugar or other sweetener has been added.

- For the ingredients list, items are provided in descending order of pre-dominance. You could buy a box of crackers, thinking it only contains sucrose (which is listed as the second item). But if you look more care-fully, you may discover that it also contains high-fructose corn syrup (the fourth ingredient), dextrose (the fifth), and molasses (the twelfth). Therefore, when you add up all these sweeteners, sugar could be the biggest item included.

- When searching for sugar, look for more than the obvious sweeteners, which end in "ose" such as sucrose, dextrose, or maltose. Visit my website, www.BeyondSugarShock.com, to get over 100 names for sugar and their definitions.

- So-called natural sugars aren't ideal, either. After all, your body will still metabolize maple syrup, barley malt, honey, and frozen fruit juice concentrates as sugars.

## Learn to Decipher Confusing Phrases on Those S.A.D. Packages

Now, it's time to learn some misleading food label claims:

- *All Natural*: This misleading term doesn't mean anything, as mentioned earlier, because the FDA has no legal standard for it.

- *Low-Fat and Fat-Free*: Reduced-fat yogurts, breads, salad dressings, or other foods may seem like healthier choices, but they may contain *as much* or *more sugar* than their high-fat

**YOU'RE A HAPPY, SUCCESSFUL SUGAR KICKER WHEN . . .**
You're turned off by S.A.D. foods with more than five ingredients.

counterparts. These products also may include potentially harmful artificial sweeteners.

- *No Added Sugar:* This term is used for foods with *naturally occurring sugars* such as in dairy products, dried fruit, tomato sauce, and other fruits or vegetables.

- *Reduced Sugar:* The FDA permits "reduced sugar" to be used on foods that contain "at least 25 percent less sugar" than leading brands. So cookies that allegedly contain "reduced sugar" may still contain a lot of sugar, even if they have 75 percent of the sugar in the original formula.

- *Sugar-Free:* These foods may contain *trace* amounts of sugar—less than .5 grams per serving. So if you have several large portions throughout the day, they still can add up to a lot of sugar.

## COACH CONNIE'S SWEET SUCCESS STRATEGY

### The Great Agave Myth: Beware!

Health-conscious people often ask me if I recommend agave syrup or agave nectar. My short answer is *No!* Unfortunately, this product is now added to many products, from energy bars to cereal products, and many health-food stores and companies often trumpet it as healthier for you, too. That's not true.

Although agave is low-glycemic, it's high in fructose, and some experts say it's worse than high-fructose corn syrup. Get more info about the provocative, much-talked-about agave at my Sugar Shock Blog.

## Skip the Sweet Fakes

It's now time to learn about the unhealthy effects of consuming what I call Sweet Fakes—i.e., those diet or low-calorie sodas, cookies, and other products filled with artificial sweeteners, such as aspartame, sucralose, saccharin, acesulfame potassium (ace-K), D-tagatose, or low-calorie sugar alcohols such as sorbitol, maltitol, mannitol, xylitol, lactitol, glycerol/glycerin, D-tagatose, isomalt, erythritol, and polydextrose.

**YOU'RE A HAPPY, SUCCESSFUL SUGAR KICKER WHEN . . .**

You tell the waiter to take away those pink, blue, and yellow packets of Sweet Fakes.

I'm opposed to Sweet Fakes for a variety of reasons. For one, drinking or eating artificially sweetened products can deplete production of serotonin (a feel-good neurotransmitter) and hence trigger cravings for carbs. That, in turn, may lead to what researchers call "paradoxical weight gain."

Just look at the stats: In 1986, about 78 million American adults used sugar-free foods and beverages, but by 2010, the number had dramatically risen, with some 194 million people consuming them, according to the Calorie Control Council, which represents the low-calorie food and beverage industry. During roughly the same time frame, obesity skyrocketed, reaching epidemic proportions.

Despite industry safety claims, Sweet Fakes aren't natural. They're what can best be described as chemical cocktails. For instance, sucralose (Splenda) contains man-made, chemically produced chlorine, which is carcinogenic; and aspartame (Equal or Nutrasweet) converts to formaldehyde, which is an embalming fluid used to preserve the dead, according to artificial sweetener expert Janet Star Hull, Ph.D., author of *Sweet Poison* and *Splenda®: Is It Safe or Not?*

Meanwhile, consumer complaints about aspartame include headaches, dizziness, memory loss, depression, and loss of libido. "The biggest reactions to Splenda include more common chlorine reactions such as skin rashes, breathing issues, bladder and kidney infections," Dr. Hull observes.

Of course, it may be overwhelming for you to think about scrapping *both* sugars *and* artificial sweeteners. But you need to know that consuming Sweet Fakes may intensify your cravings for sugary foods.

"Whatever sugar does to reinforce a sweet tooth, artificial sweeteners do even more potently," contends David Katz, M.D., M.P.H., director of the Yale-Griffin Prevention Research Center. So while you may be cutting calories in one way, "you'll likely end up consuming more calories elsewhere, because you'll crave sweeter dressings, sauces, breads, and so on."

Wouldn't it make more sense to develop an appreciation for healthy, naturally sweet foods and drinks instead?

**Affirmation: I now choose only wholesome, natural foods and beverages.**

## COACH CONNIE'S SWEET SUCCESS STRATEGY

### Begin Better with Breakfast

For generations, our parents and their parents passed on one bit of advice that many of us still ignore: "Eat breakfast." It turns out that they were right. Compelling research repeatedly reveals how vital that first meal of the day can be.

In fact, breakfast eaters "think better and faster, remember more, react quicker, are mentally sharper than skippers, [and] miss fewer days of school and work," according to nutritionist Elizabeth Somer, M.A., R.D., author of *Food & Mood.*

"Just about every measure of thinking ability improves after eating a good breakfast, from math scores and creative thinking to speed and efficiency in solving problems, concentration, recall, and accuracy in work performance."

If you skip your morning meal—as at least one-fourth of American adults do—you're setting yourself up for a big blood-sugar fall, energy slump, food cravings, and even overeating. Neglecting to have breakfast also slows your metabolism.

Eating this all-important meal also can keep your weight in check.

In fact, a Harvard study published in *Obesity*, which examined weight gain over ten years by following 20,064 U.S. men, found that, compared to breakfast eaters, breakfast skippers gained 11 pounds or more.

It's now time to plan some healthy breakfasts.

### S.A.D. to SWEET Breakfast Choices

**S.A.D.:** A cinnamon raisin bagel with a thick slab of cream cheese or a glazed donut with a glass of orange juice and two cups of coffee with 2 teaspoons of sugar.

**SWEET:** Super Oatmeal (see page 226)

2 hard-boiled, omega-3 enriched free-range eggs with yolks (3 for men or those who weigh more than 200 pounds).

**S.A.D.:** A bowl of sugary cereal, milk, a banana, and a piece of toasted white bread with lots of butter.

**SWEET:** Egg and Veggie Scramble (see page 219)

1 slice no-sugar-added, whole-grain bread such as French Meadow Healthseed Spelt Bread, Mestemacher Fitness Bread, or Food for Life's Ezekiel 4:9 100% Flourless, Organic, Sprouted Grain Bread. If you're going gluten-free, substitute with a cup of fresh fruit or 1 slice low-sugar, gluten-free bread.

1 cup sliced strawberries.

## Congratulations on Completing Week Two

In this week, you began to feed your mind positive thoughts and give your body more nourishing foods and beverages. In addition, you began to keep track of what you're putting into your lovely temple. Plus, you've decided which method works best for you to release your sugar habit, and you've mentally prepared yourself for when you do quit sweets.

It's now time for a quick review.

**YOU'RE A HAPPY, SUCCESSFUL SUGAR KICKER WHEN...**
You wonder how you used to survive on your S.A.D. breakfasts.

## Before You Head into Week Three, Have You Introduced Sweeter Habits?

- Did you start a love affair with your body and begin to give it appreciation and respect?

- Are you whispering sweet nothings to yourself every time you pass a mirror?

- Have you decided whether to quit sugar cold turkey or gradually taper off?

- Are you tracking everything you eat or drink in a notebook, or via e-mail, phone, or my Beyond Sugar Shock Food-to-Mood Tracker?

- Are you following the seven Sugar Sinning guidelines, or are you avoiding this "cheating" Adventurcise altogether, because you're a Red-Lighter around sugar?

- Do you carefully inspect food labels for such misleading terms as "all natural," "low-fat" or "fat-free," and "sugar-free"?

- Are you beginning better with breakfast and making SWEET choices?

If you've forgotten to undertake some of these activities, it's no biggie. Just start to do them now before you move into Week Three, the halfway point of *Beyond Sugar Shock*.

## CHAPTER 7

## WEEK THREE

# YOUR SPIRIT: STAY FOCUSED & HAPPY AS YOU CLEAR OUT THE NEGATIVE CLUTTER

### Affirmation: I feed my Spirit with love, gratitude, and forgiveness.

This is a pivotal point for you in the Beyond Sugar Shock program. Around the third week on a new diet or food plan, many people find that their once-strong drive has taken a nosedive. But that's not going to happen to you. Not on my watch!

That's why I've designed this week's activities to make your spirits soar and help you make lasting changes that bring you harmony, joy, and contentment. You'll wipe away disempowering thoughts, upsetting emotions, and unfinished business with your former S.A.D. ways, all of which can weigh you down or trip you up as you seek to move forward in a positive direction.

It's time to start two smart, simple, non-food-related habits. You'll get ample Vitamin Z (a good night's sleep) and begin to work out regularly (at least three to five times a week). While these are both quite powerful, effective ways to help carb cravings vanish or dissipate, they're also simple techniques to bring you inner peace and joy.

Plus, this week, you'll begin to make a major shift in consciousness. Right now, you may still feel like an embattled, frustrated sugar addict, but that will soon change. You're on your way to becoming a Spiritual Sugar Liberator like me. Soon, I predict, you'll be at the forefront of a movement to make us a nation of conscious eaters.

Now, get ready to feel relieved, refreshed, and renewed.

Week Three: **YOUR SPIRIT**
**STEP 1:** Snatch Enough Vitamin Z
**STEP 2:** Get a Natural High
**STEP 3:** Find Your Sweet Serene Spot (Meditate)
**STEP 4:** Forgive and Cleanse with Ho'oponopono & Cultivate Gratitude

## STEP 1: SNATCH ENOUGH VITAMIN Z

### Affirmation: Every night, I get as much refreshing sleep as I need.

You may be wondering why I've included information about sleep in a section dedicated to your Spirit. Well, when you're tired, cranky, unfocused, and unproductive, do you *really* feel like even trying to connect with your inner essence, or what I call your Sweet Serene Self?

On the flip side, if you've had ample shut-eye, don't you feel brighter, bouncier, and more alive? When you're well rested, don't you feel more like a child of God?

Get enough sleep and not only will your Spirit soar, but you'll become happier and more interested in cultivating a spiritual practice.

Indeed, no matter how committed, motivated, or determined you are to break free of sugar's stranglehold over you and shed weight, not getting enough sleep (or as I call it, Vitamin Z) will set you up to continually crave culprit carbs.

In short, walking around sleep deprived—something about 100 million Americans do—is a recipe for irritability, anxiety, depression, and eating inferior foods. Your body's ability to regulate hunger and fullness are controlled by the hormones leptin and ghrelin, explains James Maas, Ph.D., author of *Sleep for Success!* and *Power Sleep.*

"When you're sleep deprived, your leptin levels drop, and you don't feel as satisfied after eating. At the same time, your ghrelin levels rise, which stimulates your appetite and can make you feel starved for sugar," Dr. Maas adds, speaking on my *Gab with the Gurus Radio Show.*

Studies even show that not getting enough sleep can trigger carb cravings. For instance, researchers at Columbia University in New York City found that sleep-deprived participants ate an average of 300 more calories a day. And guess what they wanted? Ice cream and fast food.

So when you don't get enough Z's, not only do you want *more* food, but you want more of the nutrient-poor S.A.D. stuff, such as chocolate, pastries, and candies, explains Michael Breus, Ph.D., author of *The Sleep Doctor's Diet Plan: Lose Weight Through Better Sleep.*

On top of that, if you don't get your 7½ to 8½ hours of sleep (what most people need), you may have challenges concentrating, remembering things, communicating, writing clearly, making good decisions, and being creative or productive.

Research also shows that sleep deprivation can lead to a greater risk of hypertension, heart attacks, strokes, periodontal disease, and type 2 diabetes.

The good news, however, is that enough sleep can help to switch off your carb cravings and can even trigger weight loss.

"One more hour of sleep per night will let you lose, on average, a pound a week," contends Dr. Maas. "It's the best diet there is."

Sleep more, weigh less! That's *eeeeeasy!*


## Are You Craving Sleep, Not Sugar?

Take a few moments to explore your carb cravings and sugar consumption patterns so you can discover how they're related to your sleep patterns.

- At around 2 or 3 P.M. when you begin to drag, do you grab sweets (milk chocolate, soda, hard candies, etc.) or quickie carbs (chips, crackers, popcorn, etc.) on autopilot? Yes _____ No _____

- On days when you don't get enough shut-eye, do you crave more sugary or quickie-carb nonfoods? Yes _____ No _____

- Do you wake up craving high-starch carbs? Yes _____ No _____

- Do you fall asleep on the couch after watching TV and chomping on popcorn, potato chips, or cookies? Yes _____ No _____

- Do you find it easier to eat better and stay away from quickie carbs on weekends when you can catch up on sleep? Yes _____ No _____

- Do you often stay up late even though you're tired and then eat culprit carbs late at night? Yes _____ No _____

If you answered yes to one or more questions, getting the right dose of Vitamin Z may help you slam the brakes on your carb addiction so that you'll get more in control.

# RÉAL HAMILTON-ROMEO

## SWEET SUCCESS STORY

### "How I Slept My Way to Weight Loss!"

*Note from Connie: Publicist Réal Hamilton-Romeo was one of seven readers who participated in a sleep study commissioned by* Glamour *magazine and designed by "Sleep Doctor" Michael Breus, Ph.D., and Steven Lamm, M.D. Their goal: get at least 7½ hours of sleep each night, make no significant diet or exercise changes, and see if their weight changes. At the end of ten weeks, Hamilton-Romeo lost seven pounds—just by sleeping more.*

**My Sleep Habits Before the Study:** "I was averaging five to six hours of sleep each night. After the first week of the study, I was getting seven and then seven and a half hours of sleep."

**My Weight Had Plateaued:** "Before the study began, I was working out three hours a day doing cardio and strength training, but nothing was working. My weight wouldn't budge anymore. I'd lost most of the 50 pounds I'd gained when pregnant, but I had plateaued."

**I Was Known as "The Candy Store":** "At any given time, you could come by my desk at work and find a number of sweets or confections there—gummies, Laffy Taffy, Skittles, SweeTARTS—you name it, I had it. All day long, I would just sit munching on candies."

**My Candy Cravings Vanished:** "After doing the study, I threw all the candy away. I didn't want sweets anymore. I lost my taste for them. I didn't need that extra kick to keep me up during the day. Instead, I began to crave water."

**Sleep Made My Weight Slide Off:** "After six weeks of just getting enough sleep, I started to notice my pant legs get looser, and my stomach got a lot flatter. I lost seven pounds during the ten weeks. I'm 5'4" and now weigh 130."

**How Sleep Changed My Life:** "Sleep changed my disposition. I have more energy. I wake up refreshed. I spring into action in the morning. I concentrate better, and I'm more productive at work. I'm not as grumpy and grouchy. My complexion has improved. I look more vibrant. And, my *joie de vivre* came back."

**My Young Daughter Is Sold, Too:** "Before it was a chore getting her to bed at night and dragging her out of bed in the morning. But she's developed a love for wanting to go to sleep. Now, at age four, she wants her ten hours. She has more energy, her development is faster, her eating is better, and she can concentrate better."

## Tips to Get Your Rejuvenating, Slimming Vitamin Z

- *Curtail caffeine.* Don't drink coffee after 1 or 2 P.M. or within 12 hours of bedtime. "Caffeine fragments sleep, because it inhibits the neurotransmitter adenosine, which is a natural chemical you need to sleep," says Thomas Roth, Ph.D., director of research and chief of sleep medicine at Henry Ford Hospital in Detroit.

- *Bid booze bye-bye.* Ideally, you're already cutting back on alcohol because it turns to sugar, but make sure to pass up on booze three hours before bedtime.

- *Power off.* Nightfall causes your brain to produce melatonin, "a natural sleep protagonist." But if you're working on your laptop or watching TV before bedtime, the physical light decreases your melatonin levels and counteracts your brain's ability to knock you out, explains Robert Oexman, D.C., director of the Sleep to Live Institute, based in Joplin, Missouri.

**YOU'RE A HAPPY, SUCCESSFUL SUGAR KICKER WHEN . . .** Getting Vitamin Z is more important to you than opening e-mails late at night.

- *Curb your carb snacks.* If you're eating sugary foods or high-carb snacks between dinner and bedtime, they can cause you to wake up and gain weight, explains nutritionist and exercise physiologist Jill Lane, C.N.C. "Your snack will raise your blood sugar, *even if* you're asleep. That blood-sugar spike or subsequent blood-sugar low can wake you up, and you'll be hungry again."

- *Take a catnap.* If you're sleep deprived, grab a "power nap" or two of 15–20 minutes in length, recommends Dr. Maas. But don't sleep too long, because you could get groggy and later have insomnia.

- *Skip late-night dinners.* Try to eat dinner at least three hours before bedtime. Late-night eating can lead to twice as much weight gain, even if you consume *the same total calories,* according to one study from Northwestern University. (Although this study was done on mice, the results suggest that this may be true in humans, too.)

- *Set an alarm clock when it's time to go to sleep.* So suggests Dr. Michael Breus.

- *Keep a regular bedtime schedule.* Our bodies want the same sleep-wake schedule, because it strengthens our body's circadian rhythms. "If you don't keep a regular schedule, it's like you're having chronic jetlag," contends Dr. Oexman.

- *Create a cave.* Your bedroom should be dark, quiet, and cool, preferably between 67 and 70 degrees F. If your room is warmer or colder, it can cause restlessness.

- *Hit the gym earlier.* Don't exercise three to four hours before hitting the sack, because exercise makes you physically tired, not sleepy.

## Adventurcise: Personalize Your Vitamin Z Plan

What changes can you make to get enough sleep? Pick from tips offered above, and add your own.

1._____

2._____

3._____

4._____

5._____

## STEP 2: GET A NATURAL HIGH

## Affirmation: I get a soothing natural high by exercising almost every day.

Next to sleeping enough, exercise is the most important activity that can nurture and nourish your Body, Mind, and Spirit at the same time. That's why now, if you haven't already begun to do so, it's time to discover that there's absolutely nothing more invigorating, thrilling, and calming than the natural high you get from moving.

Of course, exercise is healthy for you, too, but right now your immediate goal is to do physical activities that bring you profound joy, peace of mind, bliss, spiritual contentment, pleasure, exuberance, and euphoria.

Indeed, devotees of running, bicycling, yoga, Pilates, or other workouts often say that their favorite fitness routines form a cornerstone for a spiritual practice. They say things like, *"It brings me closer to God,"* or *"It connects me to the Universe."*

For my part, Zumba, bicycling, intenSati (which you'll learn more about in Week Six), or dancing in my living room nurtures my Spirit in a way that sugar never could. Soon you'll learn what I mean.

Moving your glutes, quads, and feet can play a huge role in helping you quit eating sugar or overeating. Working out also shuts down your appestat, the mechanism in the brain that controls appetite, according to Nancy Appleton, Ph.D., author of *Suicide by Sugar.*

Of course, regular exercise also can help you shed pounds, maintain weight loss, and develop and sustain healthy bones, muscles, and joints. And working out regularly lessens symptoms of depression and anxiety, thus contributing to a happier, more balanced life.

## Exercise Less & Get More Benefits—Just Do Bursting

If you think you don't have time to work out, you're wrong. You can easily fit in exercise in *less time* by doing high-intensity interval training, also known as cardio burst training, or just bursting. In fact, this is the most effective and time-efficient way to turn your body into a fat-burning machine.

A significant body of research demonstrates the superior benefits of bursting over those slower, repetitive 20-to-60-minute workouts we've all been told to do for years. For instance, one now-famous Japanese study found that athletes who did seven or eight sprints of 20 seconds for five days a week had better aerobic capacity than athletes who did an hour of cardiovascular training on the treadmill five days a week.

"Bursting is what we humans were designed to do," explains Mark J. Smith, Ph.D., a leading authority on the health benefits of bursting. "In the Paleolithic or Stone Age era about two million years ago, when we were hunter-gatherers, we always needed to sprint to either *catch* food or not *become* food."

**YOU'RE A HAPPY, SUCCESSFUL SUGAR KICKER WHEN . . .**
Your life feels incomplete if you don't burst several times a week.

Of course, bursting gives you that all-important feel-good effect. "Cardio burst training raises feel-good chemicals, such as serotonin and dopamine, helps with better glucose tolerance, and creates less oxidative stress," explains nutrition and fitness expert JJ Virgin, Ph.D., author of *Six Weeks to Sleeveless and Sexy.*

Bursting also helps raise lactic acid, which releases human growth hormone or the hormone of youth, Dr. Virgin explains. (Lactic acid is a byproduct your body creates when you use a lot of energy quickly.)

In short, you'll get leaner, younger, and happier in less time. SWEET!

---

## How to Burst & Blast Fat from Dr. JJ Virgin

- First, warm up for three minutes.

- Then go all out—as hard as you can until you can't go a second longer—for short, intense intervals of 30–60 seconds. You can sprint/walk, cycle, jump rope, walk/run up and down stairs, swim, or use an X-iser.

- Then, recover for one to two minutes.

- Repeat until you accumulate four minutes of bursting, or eight if you're already in great shape and want to take it to the next level.

- Alternate. Burst train on one day and weight train the next, for five or six days a week.

- That's it! You're done.

---

### If You're Out of Shape . . .

If you haven't been working out in a long time, first get your doctor's okay, and then start moving. Just begin slowly—go for a walk, do yoga, and then add bursting. Initially, aim for 15–30 minutes, as often as possible, or a minimum of three days a week, recommends exercise physiologist and nutritionist Jill Lane, C.N.C.

## Adventurcise: Your Physical Activity Plan

What exercises will you do this week, when, and for how long?

Monday: _____

Tuesday: _____

Wednesday: _____

Thursday: _____

Friday: _____

Saturday: _____

Sunday: _____

## STEP 3: FIND YOUR SWEET SERENE SPOT (MEDITATE)

### Affirmation: Every day I find my Sweet Serene Spot so I can feel calm, centered, and connected to the Universe.

Now you're going to learn how to tune in to and celebrate what I playfully call your *Sweet Serene Spot*. Basically, I'm urging—no, insisting—that you start a daily spiritual practice of meditation.

When you turn inward in this manner, you quiet your mental chatter and train your mind to focus on your breathing, mantras, beautiful sounds, or feelings of compassion.

Meditation is powerful, soothing, and totally transformative. Spiritual teacher Marianne Williamson, author of the wonderful book, *A Course in Weight Loss*, says that "meditation gives us a sense of inner calm in a way that no pharmaceutical could ever do. Meditation brings the darkness to light."

What's more, meditating "helps control unwise eating or [other] acting out of compulsive behavior," Williamson explained on my *Gab with the Gurus Radio Show*.

## A Closer Look at Meditation

To get a better understanding of meditation, let's turn to one of my favorite meditation masters, Jon Kabat-Zinn, Ph.D., founder of the Center for Mindfulness in Medicine, Health Care, and Society at the University of Massachusetts Medical School.

Meditation is "an act of love, an inward gesture of benevolence and kindness toward ourselves and toward others, a gesture of the heart that recognizes our perfection even in our obvious imperfection, with all our shortcomings, our wounds, our attachments, our vexations, and our persistent habits of unawareness," Dr. Kabat-Zinn writes in his book *Coming to Our Senses*.

Healing expert Deepak Chopra, M.D., puts it another way: "Meditation is a way to get into the space between your thoughts," he said on *The Dr. Oz Show*. "According to wisdom traditions, this space between the thoughts is the window, the corridor, the vortex to the infinite mind, the mystery that some people call the spirit or God."

**YOU'RE A HAPPY, SUCCESSFUL SUGAR KICKER WHEN . . .**
You realize that quickie carbs can never fill your deep spiritual emptiness.

There, Chopra adds, you can find "a field of infinite possibilities, pure potentiality, infinite creativity, infinite imagination, and the power of intention, [which], when brought to this space, orchestrates its own fulfillment—what people call the Law of Attraction."

Of course, meditation has many other physical and emotional benefits, too. Studies show that meditating regularly can decrease your blood pressure, lower cholesterol levels, slow down your heart rate, boost your immune function, reduce production of such stress hormones as cortisol and adrenaline, promote more restful sleep, help you use oxygen more efficiently, increase production of the antiaging hormone DHEA, and even give you more gray matter in your brain—the part that's responsible for attention and mental flexibility.

In addition, meditation can help you boost self-awareness, break patterns of negative thinking, cultivate positive emotions, and be more emotionally stable.

I hope you're ready to start meditating.

## No Time to Meditate?

If your schedule is hectic, you can still squeeze meditation into your day. You can meditate while you wait in traffic, or in the waiting room of your doctor's office.

David Harp, co-author of *The Three Minute Meditator,* offers ideas on how to squeeze enriching meditation moments into your day:

**YOU'RE A HAPPY, SUCCESSFUL SUGAR KICKER WHEN . . .**

You become mindful or meditate while in line at the bank, supermarket, or post office.

- *Meditate while in line at the supermarket or bank.* "Just turn your attention onto your breath, and you'll be calm even if a stressed-out person cuts in front of you," Harp recommended during an interview on my *Gab with the Gurus Radio Show.*

- *Meditate while you walk.* "Focus on your walking, noticing, for instance, which part of your foot touches the ground first each time it hits the floor or sidewalk. At the same time, notice if you're breathing in or out."

- *Meditate en route to the fridge:* "When you're on the way from your couch to your refrigerator, count the number of steps you take for each in breath and each out breath," Harp recommends. Let us know on Facebook if you've used this cool tip!

---

### COACH CONNIE'S SWEET SUCCESS STRATEGY

## Do Yoga to Lose Weight, Cut Cravings, Unwind, and Be More Present

It's now time to strike some poses. By this, I mean start doing yoga. Originally developed centuries ago in ancient India, yoga is the original Mind-Body-Spirit exercise, and it's now popular with some 15 million Americans. Like meditation, yoga draws your attention inward.

Research now shows that yoga can help you reduce stress by lowering cortisol levels; relieve pain; curtail or stop cravings; reduce hunger; shed or maintain weight; improve psychological health; increase strength, balance, and flexibility; eat more mindfully; and get spiritually connected.

In addition to yoga, you also may wish to try other Mind-Body-Spirit practices such as Tai Chi, a gentle Chinese martial art, or Qigong, a Chinese movement exercise that literally means "cultivating energy."

## STEP 4: FORGIVE AND CLEANSE WITH HO'OPONOPONO & CULTIVATE GRATITUDE

### Affirmation: I fully and freely forgive myself for having abused my body.

The time has come to do something you may have been avoiding for years: you need to forgive yourself for wrongs you've committed against your better self, especially how you've thoughtlessly, repeatedly inhaled so much junk food. You also want to let go of grievances and grudges against other people and seek the forgiveness of others.

Not forgiving yourself or others may be why you have a sugar habit or excess weight in the first place. When you forgive, you can open your heart, strengthen your spirituality, and break out of your painful rut.

Research shows that letting go of anger, resentment, blame, and other negative emotions also relaxes muscles, lowers your blood pressure, reduces and releases stress, helps prevent heart disease, lowers cholesterol, and improves your sleep.

Releasing anger at yourself is as important, if not more important, than forgiving others, because you're taking back control.

Remember, though, that "forgiveness doesn't mean you're forgetting or denying that painful things occurred," explains Fred Luskin, Ph.D., director of the Stanford University Forgiveness Project and author of *Forgive for Good*. "[You've decided that] bad things will not ruin your life today, even though they may have spoiled your past."

Making peace with yourself and your past also paves the way for you to quietly accept your dysfunctional sugar relationship and then view both your body and food as sacred blessings. Most important, forgiveness paves the way for you to create positive changes in the present and future.

### Ho'oponopono and the Power of Forgiveness

Now, it's time to learn Ho'oponopono, a powerful forgiveness and cleansing process that's so simple you'll be shocked. All you do is repeat over and over again: *I'm sorry, please forgive me, thank you, I love you* while thinking of the Divine.

Ho'oponopono is an ancient Hawaiian technique, which was popularized in recent years by Hawaiian therapist Ihaleakala Hew Len, Ph.D., and marketing expert Joe Vitale, a star in the hit movie and book *The Secret.*

When Vitale first heard about how Dr. Hew Len healed a ward full of mentally ill criminals just by studying their charts and doing Ho'oponopono, he dismissed it as urban legend, as he recalled on my *Gab with the Gurus Radio Show.*

But Vitale became so intrigued that he tracked down Dr. Len and started studying with him. He became amazed by Ho'oponopono's powers. The two subsequently co-authored the riveting book *Zero Limits: The Secret Hawaiian System for Wealth, Health, Peace, and More.*

Now, let Ho'oponopono work more magic on *you* so you can let go of your carb habit. Joe Vitale offers the following tips:

- "First, ask yourself, *What's going on inside of me that I have caused this addiction?"*

- "Then, silently speak to the Divine, your Higher Power [or whatever you call it], and say, *'I don't know where this came from, but I don't want it anymore so help me clean it.'"*

- "Next, silently repeat: *I'm sorry, please forgive me, thank you, I love you* in whatever order feels right to you. Just repeat these phrases over and over like a prayer or mantra all throughout your day."

**YOU'RE A HAPPY, SUCCESSFUL SUGAR KICKER WHEN . . .**

You do Ho'oponopono throughout the day while thinking about your body or your sugar habit.

"The four phrases will become your new positive self-talk in your brain," adds Vitale, who was once addicted to sugar and carbs, and ultimately lost 85 pounds.

"At its heart, this process is about taking one hundred percent responsibility," he explains. "No escape clauses, no loopholes, no blaming anybody else. That's a tough one for people to get, but once they get it, there's an enormous freedom that comes from this."

## Adventurcise: Self-Forgiveness Ho'oponopono

Jot down whatever comes to mind when you silently repeat, *I'm sorry, please forgive me, thank you, I love you* while thinking about your sugar habit.

1._____

2._____

3._____

4._____

5._____

## Adventurcise: Forgiving Others Ho'oponopono

While you repeat *I'm sorry, please forgive me, thank you, I love you,* ask yourself, *Who do I need to forgive? Why?*

1._____

2._____

3._____

4._____

5._____

## Apology Letter to Loved Ones

Approach Your Loved Ones with Forgiveness in Your Heart Now it's time to ask your loved ones for forgiveness in writing. To make this easy for you, I wrote an apology letter that you can copy by hand and give to people close to you. Make sure to reach out to all those you may have alienated by your anger outbursts, crankiness, and anxiety—or what I call your off-putting Sugar Shrew or Sugar Monster behavior.

Let me caution you, though. Some people may think you're just making excuses. They may be hooked on sugar or quickie carbs themselves, and they don't understand or don't want to learn how sugar can cause strange behavior.

Given that your significant other or loved one may not acknowledge or respect your current situation, when you give them your apology letter, you also may want to give them a copy of this book and my first book, *Sugar Shock!*, which provide more background and scientific research on the subject.

But even if those close to you don't forgive you right away, rest easy. They'll come around, I believe, once they see your remarkable personality changes and other improvements. Plus, I'm convinced, the more you do Ho'oponopono, the more readily they'll accept your apology.

---

Dear _____,

I'm so sorry for any pain that I may have caused you while I was caught up in my sugar or carb addiction.

I want you to know that I'm now doing all I can to release my carb habit. In fact, I just learned that my bad sugar and carb habits may have contributed to my mood swings, crying spells, fight picking, irrational thoughts, low libido, and anything else that you've unfortunately witnessed.

Please know that I'm now seeking help to let go of this sugar addiction.

I also want to thank you so much for being there for me. I'm very grateful for your support as I begin to triumph over my sugar addiction.

Again, I'm so sorry for hurting you. Please forgive me.

I look forward to your getting to know, love, and have fun with the new, improved me.

Love,

Your Name_____

Date _____

---

## It's Time to Cultivate Gratitude, the Cousin of Forgiveness

Now that you've begun to forgive yourself and others, you'll want to practice gratitude on a regular basis. The two are actually intertwined.

"Gratitude enhances the positive, and forgiveness deletes the negative," explains psychologist and psychotherapist Philip Friedman, Ph.D., author of *The Forgiveness Solution*. "If you're grateful, the easier it is to forgive, and if you forgive, the easier it is to be grateful."

Your next assignment may seem strange. You want to *be grateful for your sugar and carb habit.* When you're grateful for *everything* that's happened to you, you see the good in it, no matter what. Plus you're shifting the focus away from yourself.

Even if you don't feel like being thankful for your sugar challenges, then consider this proof: science now shows that when you're regularly grateful, you get "higher levels of positive emotions such as joy, enthusiasm, love, happiness, and optimism," according to researcher Robert Emmons, Ph.D., author of *Thanks! How the New Science of Gratitude Can Make You Happier.*

In fact, Dr. Emmons found that people who kept gratitude journals on a weekly basis worked out more regularly, felt better about their lives, had fewer physical symptoms, and were even more optimistic about the week ahead, as opposed to people who wrote about their hassles or neutral life events. In another research project, Dr. Emmons discovered that keeping gratitude lists made people "more likely to have made progress toward important personal goals . . . over a two-month period."

Get the message? If you're grateful now, you're more likely to make progress toward your kick-sugar goal.

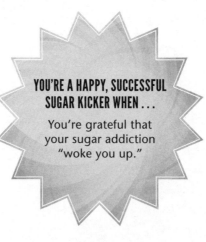

**YOU'RE A HAPPY, SUCCESSFUL SUGAR KICKER WHEN . . .**
You're grateful that your sugar addiction "woke you up."

**COACH CONNIE'S SWEET SUCCESS STRATEGY**

## Be Grateful Daily

Here are some tips to get started.

- *Keep a gratitude journal.* When things don't go as you'd like, just look at your past entries. They'll inevitably cheer you up and put a smile on your face!

- *Thank your sugar addiction.* Journal as often as you like about how your sugar addiction is a blessing.

- *Every day, say thanks for three things.* Then post your comments on my Facebook page as part of the ongoing Daily Gratitude Celebration.

- *Thank your body.* The more you appreciate your body, the more you'll love yourself, which means you'll be more inclined to eat healthy foods.

- *Start your day with a gratitude prayer.* My favorite way to start my day is with a prayer I learned years ago from a rabbi. It goes like this: *Thank you, God, for another day of life. I appreciate, God, that I am alive. I give thanks to you, oh Lord my God, that you have renewed my spirit within with great compassion and mercy.*

- *End your day saying thanks.* "Think about three wonderful things that happened during the day and say to yourself, *If the only thing that happened to me today was [fill in], it would have been enough,*" suggests Rabbi Irwin Kula, author of *Yearnings: Embracing the Sacred Messiness of Life.*

## The Power of Gratitude

As you'll soon learn, it's powerful to undertake the upcoming gratitude Adventurcise, which clients complete during my Sugar Freedom Now Course. All you do is fill in this sentence, "Today, I'm grateful for . . ."

Before you get going, first see this creative list from Judith B. of Kent, England. Here's her list:

1. Toilet paper and toilets that flush.

2. I can read and write.

3.  I can talk and listen.

4.  I can say whatever I want—I can express my own views.

5.  Computers and the Internet.

6.  I can eat.

7.  Telephones.

8.  Electricity and lightbulbs.

9.  My dog.

10. I can walk unaided.

11. I can see—nature in itself is beautiful.

Great list, isn't it? Now it's your turn.

## Adventurcise: Gratitude

Today, I'm grateful for:

1. _____

2. _____

3. _____

4. _____

5. _____

## Bonus Step: Tap Away Your Spiritual Emptiness & Anxiety

It's now time to learn another really simple, but profoundly powerful tool, called *Tapping,* or Emotional Freedom Technique (EFT), which can help you to easily release sugar cravings, and uncover and break through feelings of inadequacy, self-hate, anger, spiritual emptiness, and other issues.

Developed by Gary Craig, EFT has been hailed by myriad health and empowerment experts, who praise its remarkable effectiveness to resolve a host of conditions or ailments, including weight problems, cravings, addictions, stress, anxiety, phobias, smoking, guilt or shame, relationship blocks, low self-esteem, and allergies.

So what is it? "EFT is like psychological acupressure, but instead of an acupuncturist putting needles in you, you gently tap your fingertips on meridian points that have been used in Chinese medicine for more than 5,000 years while you focus on your cravings, conflicts, challenges, or issues and make positive statements," explains EFT master and addictions counselor David Rourke.

"This releases, smoothes, and clears the blocks in our energy system," explains EFT master Carol Look, author of *Attracting Abundance with EFT*.

Intrigued? Good! Just go to my website, www.BeyondSugarShock.com, to download your free tapping chart and an audio tapping program that guides you through a tapping sequence to help you release your sugar habit. You'll be surprised at the simplicity but effectiveness of this amazing technique.

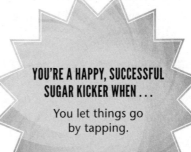

YOU'RE A HAPPY, SUCCESSFUL SUGAR KICKER WHEN . . .
You let things go by tapping.

## Bid a Final Farewell to Sweets and Welcome Sugar Shock Freedom

As we finish Part II and enter the final three weeks of the Beyond Sugar Shock program, it's natural to feel distressed, distraught, and disappointed that you have to say good-bye to your favorite sweets and carbs.

So let's take this opportunity to transform this into a special, loving, farewell ceremony, where you get rid of all the sugar-filled and processed foods in your house (or just those that belong to you, if you live with roommates or family members).

A ritual such as this is important, because it allows you "to honor the occasion, reflect on its significance to you, and then move forward so you can make a clean start," explains Barbara Biziou, author of *The Joy of Ritual* and *The Joys of Family Rituals*.

Before you toss out your favorite junk foods, first thank them for serving you and giving you comfort, Biziou recommends.

Now ditch those culprit carbs with pomp and ceremony and a feeling of finality and victory. Make sure to toss them down the garbage chute or put them in a recycling container or bin, on the curb so you can't retrieve them later—something many sugar addicts admit to me that they've done in moments of weakness.

Next, cleanse your home of negative energy. Just light a candle, burn incense or sage, listen to calming music, and open the door of your home to welcome in new energy, Biziou suggests.

Enjoy your newfound, intoxicating, euphoric feeling of Sugar Shock Freedom.

Now, before you begin the second half of your Beyond Sugar Shock program, make sure to go shopping for some healthy foods. Just go to the back of the book to get your shopping list, and either bring this book with you on your expedition or make a copy to bring to the farmers' market and/or supermarket.

## Did Your Spirits Begin to Lift in Week Three?

Hurrah for you! You've reached an important point. You've now completed half of your Beyond Sugar Shock program.

This week, you finished laying the foundation for your sugar-free success by devoting attention to pursuing activities and practices that lift your spirits. It's now time to take a look back at what you learned and to review your new, smart, Spirit-filling habits.

## Before You Head into Week Four, Have You Renewed Your Spirit?

- Are you getting enough of the satisfying, replenishing Vitamin Z every night? Note in your journal how much better you now feel.

- Are you bursting, doing strength training, or getting other regular exercise at least three days a week?

- Are you discovering your Sweet Serene Spot by meditating every day?

- Are you doing Ho'oponopono (simply privately saying, *I'm sorry, please forgive me, thank you, I love you*) throughout your day?

- Did you give your loved ones your apology letter?

- Are you keeping a gratitude journal?

- Are you posting three things for which you're thankful on my Facebook page?

- Did you copy your Beyond Sugar Shock Shopping List and bring it with you to buy healthy foods?

- How have you found that focusing on your Spirit this week took away some of your desire for sweets? Write about it in your journal.

It's time for me to applaud you. You're now ready to move into the final three-week phase of *Beyond Sugar Shock*.

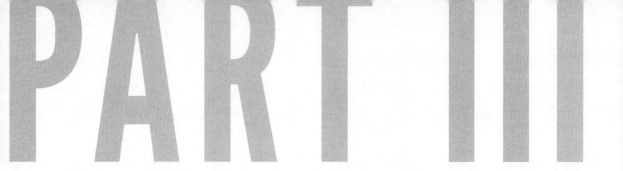

# PART III

# YOUR LAST
# THREE WEEKS

YOUR SWEETER LIFE BEGINS

## CHAPTER 8

## WEEK FOUR

# YOUR BODY: PUT YOUR PLAN INTO ACTION BY EATING WHOLESOME, SWEETERLICIOUS FOODS

**Affirmation: I now release my addiction to sugar and other nutrient-lacking, fake foods. I desire only real, health-giving, nutritious foods. I accept perfect health and my ideal weight now.**

Are you ready for what could be the most transformational time of your life? As we begin Part III of this Beyond Sugar Shock program, it's time for you to discover the absolutely remarkable, formidable, life-changing power of letting go of your reliance on those nutrient-robbed, processed sweets and quickie carbs.

Last week, in your farewell ceremony, you said *So long, enough already* to your health-harming S.A.D. habits. This week, you're bidding a warm *Hello* to nourishing, health-giving, mood-lifting, confidence-building foods and a sweeterlicious life.

Specifically, this week you're putting your very own personalized Beyond Sugar Shock plan into action. You'll either quit cold turkey or cut back slowly on your intake of sugar and refined carbs.

If removing sweets and culprit carbs from your diet still feels overwhelming to you, let me reassure you that you can do it. You're *completely ready*. After all, you've been carefully preparing for this for the past three weeks.

## Your New Way of Eating: Juicy, Tasty, Satisfying Quality Carbs & Real Foods Await

Today, if you haven't already, stock up on real, quality, nourishing, nutrient-dense foods, which you'll soon discover are far tastier than those refined, fiber-stripped fake foods. Simply copy your Beyond Sugar Shock Shopping List and take it with you to Whole Foods or another quality grocery store in your area. Look for the ingredients you'll need to prepare SWEET, sugar-free recipes that are part of the book's Meal Plan.

Of course, your Beyond Sugar Shock Shopping List can guide you, but here are some helpful tips on how to buy quality foods:

- Make sure to get fresh, flavorful, nourishing, alive, preferably local, organic foods that grow out of the ground or come from trees. Or choose from well-treated, free-range animals that graze pastures or fish that have been checked for mercury content. (See my website for sources.)

- As much as possible, bypass those processed pseudo-foods, which come in jars, cans, bottles, or packages.

- Avoid prepared foods that contain more than five ingredients. There are a few exceptions to this rule—which you can find at my website.

- Ignore those tempting, treacherous center aisles, checkout stands, and places where cookies, cakes, pretzels, other quickie carbs, sweetened protein bars, and gooey concoctions are attractively displayed to entice you.

*"Let food be thy medicine and medicine be thy food."*

—HIPPOCRATES, GREEK PHYSICIAN AND THE FATHER OF MEDICINE

## How to Leave S.A.D. Behind & Plan Your SWEET, Sugar-Free Meals

You're now ready to become a Conscious Quality Eater. You'll begin to follow an anti-inflammatory diet that's a cross between a Mediterranean diet and a Paleolithic diet (the Caveman Diet or Stone Age Diet). That's how our hunter-gatherer ancestors ate for two million years, up until about 10,000 years ago when the Agricultural

Revolution began, technological innovations came of age, and food focus shifted from meat to grains.

Always keep your home filled with a variety of fiber-filled, multicolored (ideally certified organic or noncertified organic) vegetables; low-glycemic fruits, nuts, seeds, and legumes; lean grass-fed meat; superior fats; and wild fish; as well as whole grains and dairy products, if your body can handle them.

## How to Eat & Plan Your SWEET, Sugar-Free Meals

Let's start this week off right! In addition to the helpful, healthy-eating pointers I'll outline in this chapter, I've given you one week of direction on how to incorporate this new way of eating into your life. Refer to the Meal Plan on page 208 to help guide you as you make this shift. Just remember, a good rule of thumb for healthy eating is to always choose a mix of superior proteins, fats, and carbs like veggies or fruits.

For instance, at lunch and dinner, about half of your plate will come from veggies or fruits, with some legumes. A fourth will feature quality protein sources (the size of a deck of cards or the palm of your hand) and the other fourth will come from omega-3 and other smart fats such as avocado, nuts, and seeds, according to nutrition consultant and exercise physiologist Jill Lane, C.N.C., who prepared the Beyond Sugar Shock Meal Plan.

For those of you who rarely cook, don't fret. Sure, it may be new for you to prepare meals with attention, love, joy, and fresh ingredients, but soon, you'll enjoy cooking—and especially eating—meals that are not only delicious, but easy to prepare. Of course, you also can be creative and spontaneous when you create your meals. In fact, soon I expect to hear from you budding natural foods chefs. Just post your tasty recipes on the Facebook SmartHabitsFans page and in the SparkPeople Beyond Sugar Shock Freedom Team.

It's time to get cracking with specifics on smart food choices you can make to nourish your special temple. So here are this week's four steps.

Week Four: **YOUR BODY**
**STEP 1:** Party with the Produce
**STEP 2:** Pump Up the Protein
**STEP 3:** Fancy the Fats
**STEP 4:** Wipe Out the Whites—Go Whole Grain (or Not)

## STEP 1: PARTY WITH THE PRODUCE

### Affirmation: I'm now happily choosing only wholesome, colorful veggies and fruits, which bring me good health and moods.

It's now time to begin relishing Mother Nature's succulent, mouthwatering, flavorful carb gifts. Indeed, once you begin eating juicy cherry tomatoes, crunchy Kirby cucumbers, zesty red peppers, luscious Red Delicious apples, savory Bosc pears, melt-in-your-mouth avocadoes, delicious jicama, scrumptious sweet potatoes, tasty carrots, and more, you'll find that they're much more delicious and satisfying than the nutrient-deprived, health-robbing, S.A.D. foods you've been consuming until now.

### YOU'RE A HAPPY, SUCCESSFUL SUGAR KICKER WHEN ...

Your once S.A.D.-hooked child pulls you by the hand to the apples at the farmers' market and says, "Mom, can we buy some, please?"

### Take the Organic Plunge

Now that you're experimenting with fruits and veggies, you may be wondering if it's best to buy organic produce. The short answer is yes. Not only do these foods taste better, but some studies attest to the fact that organic produce is far healthier, because organic farmers don't use potentially harmful pesticides found in commercially grown food.

Organic foods contain more nutrients, vitamins, and micronutrients than commercially grown foods. One four-year European study found that organic fruits and vegetables contained up to 40 percent more antioxidants and had higher levels of iron and zinc. In fact, the differences between conventionally and organically grown produce were so marked that you could eat less than the recommended five portions a day of fruits and vegetables and still get ample nutrients.

Research suggests that a predominantly organic diet appears to lower the incidence of common conditions and diseases, such as cancer, coronary heart disease, allergies, and hyperactivity in children.

When you go organic, you also reduce the amount of toxic chemicals, food additives, and artificial colorings you ingest, and you tend to avoid those potentially toxic GMOs (genetically modified organisms).

More than 600 active chemicals are reportedly registered for agricultural use in America today. Each year, U.S. agriculture uses 1.2 billion pounds of chemical pesticides, leading each American to consume an estimated 5 pounds of chemical pesticides, according to chef and educator Ann Cooper, known as the "Renegade Lunch Lady."

Organic foods are especially important for our nation's children. While pesticides can cause neurological damage in both adults and children, research indicates that children experience a disproportionate amount of harm. So the fewer pesticides, the better.

## COACH CONNIE'S SWEET SUCCESS STRATEGY:

### Be Smart About Organics

If you're concerned that organic fruits and vegetable are too expensive, don't worry. You're getting some buying help from the Environmental Working Group (EWG), a nonprofit organization, which has compiled two lists to help you, "The Dirty Dozen" and "The Clean 15." The Dirty Dozen includes fruits and vegetables that when grown organically can reduce toxins found in them by as much as 80 percent. The Clean 15 list tells you which fruits and vegetables are lowest in toxic pesticides, even if they're not organic.

| THE DIRTY DOZEN | THE CLEAN 15 |
|---|---|
| 1. Apples | 1. Onions |
| 2. Celery | 2. Sweet corn |
| 3. Strawberries | 3. Pineapple |
| 4. Peaches | 4. Avocado |
| 5. Spinach | 5. Asparagus |
| 6. Nectarines (imported) | 6. Sweet peas |
| 7. Grapes (imported) | 7. Mangoes |
| 8. Sweet bell peppers | 8. Eggplant |
| 9. Potatoes | 9. Cantaloupe – domestic |
| 10. Blueberries (domestic) | 10. Kiwi |
| 11. Lettuce | 11. Cabbage |
| 12. Kale/collard greens | 12. Watermelon |
| | 13. Sweet potatoes |
| | 14. Grapefruit |
| | 15. Mushrooms |

Source: The Environmental Working Group.

## Put More Color on Your Plate

As you give produce a top spot in your daily menu, follow the rainbow. For instance, make sure to introduce multicolored fruits such as blackberries, blueberries, cranberries, and raspberries. "Studies show that blueberries have a positive effect on your brain chemistry, and they improve mood and cognitive performance. And cranberries are highly oxidative, meaning they mop up lots of unwanted free radicals," explains nutritionist Oz Garcia, Ph.D., whose clients include celebrities such as Oscar winner Hilary Swank.

Your best bet is to eat vegetables at every meal. You can even add veggies to your omelet in the morning. (Some tasty options include spinach, asparagus, zucchini, red and yellow peppers, broccoli, or kale.)

Colorful veggies are rich in vitamins, minerals, and antioxidants. "They also increase your fiber, move fat out of storage and into your stools, move waste through your digestive system, and deliver active compounds called phytochemicals, which may fight cancer, chronic diseases, and aging," Dr. Garcia adds.

### Coach Connie's SWEET Success Strategy

### Freeze Away Cravings—Turn Fruit into "Candy"

Naturally, during your first few days off sugar, you may crave something sweet. So try some fun food. Just pop low- or medium-glycemic fruits such as strawberries, blueberries, raspberries, blackberries, grapes, cherries, or even small slices of a peach, plum, or pear into your freezer.

Then, when you get an urge for dessert, nosh on them like candies. But when you have these sweet treats, make sure to eat some protein and/or fat at the same time, such as a few nuts, a slice of goat cheese, or a tablespoon of sugar-free almond butter. Scrumptious!

# FELICIA DESROSIERS

## "How Veggies Helped Me Become Sugar-Free"

*Note from Connie: When I attended the Institute for Integrative Nutrition, I met Felicia Desrosiers (www.HolisticCounsel.org), and we instantly bonded over our shared previous sugar addiction. Here is her story.*

**Sugar Was My Reward:** "I remember as a child being given a big jar of hard candies after being brave—and this was from *my dentist!* I learned at a young age that candy—sugar—was a reward."

**I Was Sick All the Time:** "Over the years, I had a stomach ulcer (at age 10, no less), cysts, terrible PMS, borderline anemia, acne, water retention, recurring gastritis, irritable bowel syndrome, allergies, congestion, chronic fatigue, depression, insomnia, and bloating. Plus, I was on a permanent emotional roller coaster, and I felt stuck in my life. I wish someone had told me that sugar was causing most of my problems. I cut out sugar for good in 2001, and my life changed forever. One by one, all my symptoms went away."

**Benefits of Kicking Sugar:** "I became motivated, focused, and happier, as well as more energetic, productive, and creative. In addition, my digestion improved, and my constipation and congestion vanished. Plus, the emotional roller-coaster rides and bouts of depression disappeared, and my relationships got better. And, five to seven unwanted pounds just slipped right off without my even trying."

**Veggies Helped Me Quit Sugar:** "When giving up sugar, I found it crucial to eat sweet vegetables, squash, plantains, green leafy vegetables, and whole grains on a daily basis. They helped change my taste buds and made refined sugary foods too sweet."

## Adventurcise: Party with the Produce

It's now time to take what you've learned and put it into action.

**What fruits and veggies will you try this week?**

1._____

2._____

3._____

4._____

5._____

**Come back after you eat them.**

**What were your favorites? Why?**

1._____

2._____

3._____

4._____

5._____

**Were you surprised by how sweet some fruits and veggies tasted?**

Yes _____ No _____ If so, which ones?

_____

**Thoughts/Conclusions**

_____

_____

COACH CONNIE'S SWEET SUCCESS STRATEGY

## Beware of Dates & Other Dried Fruits

Watch out for high-glycemic dried fruits, which cause spikes of glucose or sugar in your blood. Some clients say that if they have a few pieces of dates or dried mangos, they want the whole bag. So be careful. And always soften the blood-sugar whammy with a few nuts or some other protein-fat combo.

## Winning with Water

One way to get healthier is to make sure you get ample water, an important health habit about half of Americans ignore. Not drinking enough $H_2O$ leads to dehydration, which can lead to inflammation and even premature aging.

Water makes up about 60 to 70 percent of an adult's weight, making it the single most abundant substance in the human body. However, we regularly lose water when we breathe, sweat, urinate, and have bowel movements.

Now bear in mind when I say water, I don't mean sugar-loaded, vitamin-filled "waters." Skip these S.A.D. dangers.

Drinking pure water—preferably run through some kind of filter—can keep you young, help your organs and cells function, improve your circulation, make your skin more radiant, flush waste from your cells, and help those pounds slide right away.

In fact, drinking half your body weight in ounces per day can help to prevent you from overeating, according to Ann Louise Gittleman, Ph.D., C.N.S., author of *Fat Flush for Life*. In other words, if you weigh 135 pounds, consume 67.5 ounces of water per day.

Often people who overeat really need to be drinking more water, Dr. Gittleman observes. "And as we get older, the 'thirst' trigger can become misinterpreted as the need to eat."

Here's another simple water diet trick from Drs. Michael and Mary Dan Eades, authors of *Protein Power*. Drink a large glass of cold water 15 to 30 minutes before a meal, which will reduce your hunger so you eat less. Not only that, but just drinking a glass or two of water can cut back on those pesky sugar cravings.

## Coach Connie's SWEET Success Strategy

### Spruce Up Your Water

The next time you're hungry, headachy, weak, or tired, ask yourself how much water you've been drinking. These are all signs of dehydration. You may also have dry or itchy skin, dark-colored urine, chills, and lapses in concentration.

Sip water throughout the day, perhaps every half hour. If you're drinking one-half of your body weight in ounces of water, as suggested above, most of you will have 9 to 12 eight-ounce glasses of water per day.

Add a slice of orange, lime, lemon, or cucumber; mint leaves; or a leaf of stevia to make your water more enticing. Or place a few cooked cranberries or goji berries into a tea infuser.

You can even sprinkle in some cinnamon, ginger, or clover or add a teabag of licorice, ginger, or Indian spice into your water that's either chilled or at room temperature.

And when you dine out or "have drinks" with friends, ask for sparkling water with lime or lemon instead of alcohol. In other words, make drinking water into a celebratory occasion.

**Affirmation: I now happily drink half my weight in ounces of water every day.**

### Adventurcise: Fall in Love with Water

How much water did you drink today? _____

Did you notice any changes in appetite, desire for sweets, etc., by drinking more water?

Yes _____ No _____

Explain

_____

How are you keeping track of your water intake to make sure you have enough?

_____

Thoughts/Conclusions

_____

_____

## STEP 2: PUMP UP THE PROTEIN

## Affirmation: I'm now getting enough quality protein for my body.

You may be wondering what protein has to do with your sugar habit. Actually, quite a bit.

Think about it: On days when you've gone overboard on sweets and simple carbs, how much protein did you eat before, during, and afterward? Did you skimp on the good stuff and go hog wild on the junk?

In fact, whenever you *think* you have a sugar craving, you may be deficient in healthy proteins and fats. Adding these foods can help stabilize your blood sugar. Here are some other useful facts about protein, which are abundant in fish, poultry, beef, beans, nuts, seeds, and eggs:

- *Protein curbs your hunger so you don't overeat and snack too much between meals.* Protein keeps you feeling full longer than carbs because it takes longer to break down in your body. For instance, in one study from French researchers, high-carb snackers got hungry as quickly as subjects who had no snacks at all. But protein eaters, who snacked on chicken, stayed full nearly 40 minutes longer.

- *Protein boosts your metabolism and helps you lose weight.*

- *Protein isn't stored as fat the way carbs are.* In fact, "it's very difficult and inefficient for [your body] to store excess protein as fat," points out Loren Cordain, Ph.D., author of *The Paleo Diet.*

- *Protein improves your insulin and glucose levels.* Leading metabolic researchers have found that protein-rich diets can improve long-term insulin sensitivity.

- *Protein keeps your blood sugar stable.*

- *Protein, when eaten with a higher-carbohydrate food, can help give you a smaller rise in blood glucose after your meals.*

- *Protein helps build, maintain, and repair your muscles and tissues.*

- *Protein maintains or improves mood.*

- *Protein builds strong bones.*

- *Protein boosts your immune system.*

- *Protein is needed for the growth and maintenance of our cells.*

- *Protein helps keep your hair, skin, and fingernails healthy.*

## How Much Protein Is Enough?

While you calculate your protein needs, think of protein as your powerful partner to help you break free of your sugar habit. Therefore, you should add some form of protein to every meal or snack.

But how much is enough? "Most people will do fine with having around 30 percent protein," nutritionist and weight-loss expert Jonny Bowden, Ph.D., C.N.S., explains. Of course, your individual needs vary, depending on your activity level, your body composition, metabolic type, stress level, age, and sex.

When determining how much protein to eat, you also want to take into consideration such factors as pregnancy, insulin resistance, or kidney disease. Higher protein levels *won't* cause kidney problems, but they will exacerbate them, so make sure you have no impairment in kidney function if you eat high amounts of protein, recommends Dr. Bowden, author of *Living Low Carb: Controlled-Carbohydrate Eating for Long-Term Weight Loss*.

COACH CONNIE'S SWEET SUCCESS STRATEGY

### Try This SWEET Anti-Pig-Out Insurance Policy

Before you go out to a function, dinner, or even grocery shopping, try to have a little protein snack with some raw veggies first. You may discover that the breadbasket and hors d'oeuvres, which used to be your downfall, simply lose their appeal. Not only that, but you'll be less likely to grab cookies, candies, and crackers off supermarket shelves.

Here are some preparty snacks you can try:

- A small (approximately one ounce) piece of leftover chicken with some celery or cauliflower

- A small (one ounce) portion of goat cheese with veggies or some low-glycemic fruit

- Six almonds, walnuts, or macadamia nuts

- A few pieces of raw broccoli with hummus or a hardboiled egg

- A small cup of lentil soup

## Adventurcise: Eating Protein

What protein did you have today?

Breakfast_____

Lunch _____

Dinner_____

Snack #1_____

Snack #2_____

After you ate a meal or snacks that contained protein, did you:

Feel fewer cravings for sweets? Yes _____ No _____

Feel less hungry and more satisfied? Yes _____ No _____

Go longer between meals? Yes _____ No _____

Thoughts/Conclusions

_____

_____

## Adventurcise: Eating Protein

Think about some quality sources of protein that you can enjoy this week and next. To get ideas, turn to the Beyond Sugar Shock Shopping List. Below, list your ten favorite sources of protein:

1._____

2._____

3._____

4._____

5._____

6._____

7._____

8._____

9._____

10._____

## STEP 3: FANCY THE FATS

## Affirmation: I'm now eating modest amounts of healthy fats and losing weight.

First, let's dispense with perhaps the biggest diet myth of all: much as you may have been brainwashed to be fat-phobic, you need to know that *eating fat does not make you fat.* Rather, the *right fats* can help peel off pounds and act as potent anti-inflammatory agents.

In particular, omega-3 fats, a group of polyunsaturated fatty acids, are "anti-obesity fats, which stimulate your body's metabolic ability to burn fat," according to weight-loss and detox expert Ann Louise Gittleman, Ph.D., author of *Fat Flush for Life.*

Quality fats can also help tame your sweet tooth. Essentially, fats work as "sugar stoppers that slow down the speed with which your stomach does its job on carbs," explains cardiologist Arthur Agatston, M.D. in *The South Beach Diet.*

All fats, whether they're superior or not, slow down the release of foods from your stomach into your intestines and don't give you a "sugar rush." However, for your purposes, you want to pick waist-trimming fats such as olive oil, avocado, and flaxseed oil.

## Choose Quality Omega-3 Fats

Your goal is to boost your intake of healthy fats, or essential fatty acids (EFAs). Since our bodies can't make omega-3s, we need to find them in foods we eat— from cold-water fish such as salmon, sardines, trout, halibut, mackerel, herring, and shrimp; vegetable sources such as olives and avocados; and certain nuts and seeds such as flax seeds, chia seeds, walnuts, almonds, and macadamia nuts.

A number of research studies have shown that not only can omega-3 fats help facilitate weight loss, but they can also regulate blood sugar and help prevent insulin resistance.

They can also improve your heart health; protect against cancer, rheumatoid arthritis, and other diseases; lower your cholesterol and triglyceride levels; maintain healthy skin; help reduce PMS and prevent postmenopausal symptoms; sharpen your memory; improve your moods; and even prevent or reduce depression. In short, the findings about omega-3s are pretty impressive.

## Discover the Joys of Flax, Chia Seeds, Cacao Beans, Nuts & Other Super Foods

As you seek to add different flavors and textures to your foods, I urge you to experiment with a variety of nutritional powerhouses such as flax seeds, which are rich in omega-3 fats, an excellent source of fiber, and a rich source of lignan, a plant compound shown to act in humans like a weak form of estrogen. They may also help regulate blood glucose levels and reduce the risk of heart disease and cancer.

For a crisp, nutty flavor, sprinkle ground flax seeds on your vegetable or fruit salad, lentil soup, steamed veggies, cooked cereal, fruit or plain yogurt, or soup.

You can also try fiber-rich chia seeds. Once considered a sacred Aztec and Mayan food, this vegetarian superfood is rich in omega-3 fatty acids, antioxidants, vitamin C, protein, and even minerals such as calcium, phosphorus, potassium, manganese, copper, molybdenum, and zinc.

Make sure to taste nutrient-dense raw cacao beans, too—that's real chocolate without sugar—as well as such superfoods as goji berries (in moderation), wild bee pollen, or maca.

By the way, many mornings or before a workout, I'll blend chia seeds, raw cacao beans, ground flax seeds, a pea protein or rice protein powder, Moringa, a pinch of powdered stevia and cinnamon, and some blueberries to create a nutritionally packed, tasty Chia-Cacao-Cinnamon-Stevia Shake. (Get the recipe on my Sugar Shock Blog.)

You also can liven up your favorite dishes by sprinkling on finely ground almonds, pine nuts, hazelnuts, macadamia nuts, pecans, walnuts, or even hemp seeds, which are loaded with essential amino acids and essential fatty acids.

## Avoid Health-Harming Trans Fats

As you choose more healthy omega-3 fats, make sure to cut back—or completely eliminate—health-harming, man-made *trans-fatty acids* (*trans fats*), which can increase your risk of coronary heart disease.

You can find these dangerous fats in S.A.D. foodstuffs such as fried, commercially baked foods, and fast foods. But, of course, since you're eliminating or drastically cutting back on these packaged foods anyway, you'll naturally be avoiding trans fats.

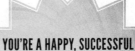

**YOU'RE A HAPPY, SUCCESSFUL SUGAR KICKER WHEN . . .**
You get excited that Whole Foods or another favorite health food store has a sale on chia seeds or flax seeds.

Here's one quick tip on how to avoid trans fats: never eat anything with the words *hydrogenated* or *partially hydrogenated* on the label. Most trans fat is formed when hydrogen is added to vegetable oil—a process called *hydrogenation*—and the liquid oils are made into solid fats such as hard margarine or shortening.

You'll also want to try to limit your intake of saturated fats, found in fatty red meats, full-fat dairy products, lard, and butter.

## Adventurcise: Eat Healthy Fats

What healthy fats will you experiment with this week? (Examples: flax oil, olive oil, fish oil, chia seeds, and coconut oil, as well as foods such as avocadoes, walnuts, macadamia nuts, almonds, salmon, shrimp, sardines, etc.)

- _____

- _____

- _____

- _____

- _____

(Fill out after eating your meals with fats.)

Did you:

Feel fewer cravings for sweets after eating meals with healthy fats? Yes ___ No ___

Feel less hungry and more satisfied? Yes _____ No _____

Eat less? Yes _____ No _____

Wait longer between meals? Yes _____ No _____

Thoughts/Conclusions

_____

_____

## Coconut Oil: The Miraculous Exception

Although you want to cut back on saturated fats, you may still want to choose organic, unrefined extra-virgin coconut oil. Research suggests that coconut oil has been shown to promote weight loss; reduce your risk of cancer, atherosclerosis, and other degenerative conditions; help prevent bacterial, viral, and fungal (including yeast) infections; support your immune system function; prevent osteoporosis; support healthy metabolic function; improve digestion and nutrient absorption; and keep your skin soft and smooth.

Coconut oil also is "one of the most stable oils for cooking—and for blood-sugar regulation," says nutritionist Ann Louise Gittleman, Ph.D.

### STEP 4: Wipe Out the Whites. Make Sweet Switcheroos. Go Whole Grain—Or Not.

## Affirmation: Refined white carbs are boring! I prefer tasty Quality Carbs.

While you're getting sugar and carbs out of your system, you can make some Sweet Switcheroos to ease the transition. In other words, replace dangerous, refined, nutrient-poor, quickly digested desserts, cereals, breads, and white rice with Mother Nature's carb gifts.

It's just as easy—and certainly more nutritious—to chomp on an apple or pear with some nut butter, or celery sticks or cauliflower chunks with homemade hummus, than to unthinkingly grab French fries or hot dogs on white buns.

Granted, it may take time for your palate to adjust, but soon you'll discover that veggies, fruits, and whole grains have a much more satisfying, clean taste than those fake nonfoods. Frankly, I don't know how I used to eat all that white-carb crap!

### Bring on the Whole Grains

To begin making sweet switcheroos, start replacing nutrient-stripped refined carbs with whole grains, such as quinoa, brown rice, amaranth, barley, buckwheat, bulgur, wheat berries, or teff, all of which release sugars in a slower, steadier, gentler manner.

Make sure any grains you eat are whole and as unprocessed as possible, because any refining removes both fiber and nutrients. The fiber retards the conversion of starch into sugar, contains no calories, and has beneficial bulk, which fills you up and satisfies your appetite while slowing your blood-sugar swings at the same time.

In fact, our bodies weren't designed to eat our modern, grain-glutted diets, say a number of scientists, nutritionists, and medical professionals. Humanity didn't become dependent upon cereal grains until the advent of the agricultural revolution a mere 10,000 years ago—a nanosecond of the time that we humans have inhabited the earth. Before that, for more than two million years, our hunter-gatherer ancestors rarely, if ever, consumed grains.

By eating so many processed grains, sugary foods, and dairy products, experts say we're more likely to develop the diseases of modern civilization such as obesity, diabetes, heart disease, and cancer. In fact, many people function just fine without grains.

## COACH CONNIE'S SWEET SUCCESS STRATEGY

### Find Out If You Have a Gluten Allergy or Sensitivity

Before you start eating a lot of grains, it's wise to find out if you suffer from gluten sensitivity or the more serious celiac disease, an inherited autoimmune disorder.

Gluten is an elastic protein and common allergen that's contained in wheat, rye, barley, spelt, kamut, triticale, farina, and often in oats (through contamination during growing, transporting or processing).

Like sugar, gluten is found in most cereals, breads, chips, crackers, pasta, and cookies, as well as in soy sauce, soups, beer, caramel flavorings, and candies.

Recent research suggests that celiac disease, an autoimmune disorder once considered rare, now afflicts one of every 133 people, according to the National Foundation for Celiac Awareness, but a whopping 97 percent of those with the problem go *undiagnosed*.

As many as 250 ailments may be linked to celiac disease or gluten sensitivity, author and "Gluten-Free Guru" Danna Korn says, citing weight gain or weight loss, fatigue, weakness, joint pain, headaches, migraines, depression, infertility, irregular menstrual cycle, anxiety, autism, gastrointestinal problems, schizophrenia, mood changes, loss of coordination, muscle cramping, and anemia.

If you suspect you have celiac disease or gluten intolerance, see a physician. Or, just try a gluten-elimination diet to see if any of your symptoms disappear.

Even if you don't have gluten issues, it can be helpful to limit your intake of all grains—even whole grains—and begin to embrace gluten-free foods instead.

## Adventurcise: It's White-Out Time!

**If you plan on eating whole grains, which ones will you choose?** These are gluten-free grains: amaranth, brown rice, buckwheat, millet, oats and oat groats (if designated gluten-free), quinoa, sorghum, teff, and products from corn or beans.

1. _____

2. _____

3. _____

4. _____

5. _____

**Now, write about your whole grain experience.**

Were you surprised how sweet these grains tasted? Yes _____ No _____

Which ones? _____

**Thoughts/Conclusions**

_____

_____

**Affirmation: If and when I snack, I always do so mindfully.**

## To Snack or Not to Snack?

People often ask me, *"Should I snack or not? And if so, what?"* Experts are divided on the issue, especially when it comes to weight loss.

Personally, I'm a big fan of smart snacking, because you won't feel deprived or ravenously hungry.

Ultimately, it's up to you to decide if you want to snack. But here are some tips to make sure you put your best food forward:

- Never skip meals, and don't go longer than four hours between eating. Otherwise, you may become so hungry that you frantically grab something bad for you.

- Create snacks that have a good mix of lean protein, fiber-rich, low-glycemic complex carbs (like vegetables and fruits), and quality fats. Protein and fat will make you feel full longer, and the fiber in the slow, superior carbs takes longer to digest. Remember, though, we're talking small portions for your snacks—these are not meals.

- Don't snack two to three hours before bedtime unless you have hypoglycemia, in which case have a small snack.

- Always keep track of snacks in your food journal.

- Beverages count. So pay attention to what you might be putting in your tea or coffee.

- Plan snacks in advance. That way, you can take a serving or two with you when you leave home.

- If you're stumped on what to have for a snack, just divide your breakfast, lunch, or dinner in half and eat the other half later as a snack. This is one of my favorite ways to quickly create foods to eat on the run, especially before or after a workout.

- Skip processed, sugary, salty, fatty snacks, especially ones from vending machines.

- Don't make impulsive snack decisions while you're in line at the drugstore or corner market. Get a list of snack ideas later in your Meal Plan.

---

**COACH CONNIE'S SWEET SUCCESS STRATEGY**

### *On the Side, Please* When You Dine Out

Although you're nixing the culprit carbs, you can still stay sweetly sugar-free while dining out. My best advice is encapsulated in the words, *On the side, please.*

No matter where you are—in a nice, candlelit restaurant or brightly lit dining establishment—always politely and sweetly ask for all sauces, salad dressings, or toppings *on the side, please*. You might feel uncomfortable at first, but trust me, your servers are used to such requests.

If you like, you can even dip your fork lightly into the sauce to take a taste, or ask for lemon or olive oil to add some zest to your meal.

## Other Tips to Dine Out with Ease

Here are a few more tips to help stick to your sugar-free diet while dining out.

- *Do homework first.* Before you head out to a restaurant, peek at the menu online or call in advance to make sure you'll have plenty of quality, fiber-rich veggies and other sugar-free options.

- *Banish the breadbasket.* If you're with health-conscious diners, ask if they'd be willing to skip the breadbasket at your table. If not, then make sure those tempting white carbs are on *the other side of the table.*

- *Veggie up and pick polite portions.* Whenever possible, especially for dinner or lunch, order a large salad; a palm-sized portion of lean protein such as chicken, fish or turkey; and a vegetable side dish. And be sure to drink eight ounces of water.

- *Skip salt.* Unless the restaurant carries sea salt, it's smart to ask your server to tell the chef to skip the salt.

- *Pass on the alcohol.* When dining out, try to avoid wine, beer, or other alcohol, which can trigger cravings and overeating.

Now relax, enjoy your meal and your wonderful company, and have fun.

## How Does It Feel to Bless, Respect, & Appreciate Your Body by Giving It Quality Foods?

For Week Four of *Beyond Sugar Shock*, you got a lot of valuable information about what kinds of foods to eat, along with simple ideas about the types of foods that will make your body function at its best.

Remember, I'm not advocating that you go low-carb—that is, unless you want to. Rather, I'm urging you to choose Quality Carbs as often as possible.

As you introduce new, better food practices, you'll easily, effortlessly transform your body into a slimmer, fat-burning machine. Not only that, but as you feed yourself smart foods, you'll become smarter, quicker, happier, and sweeter.

Now, it's time for a quick recap.

## Before You Head into Week Five, Have You Changed the Way You Eat?

- At lunch and dinner, are you filling your plate with fresh, fiber-rich veggies?

- Have you been trying vegetables and fruits from all colors of the rainbow?

- Are you making sure to consume quality protein, which can reduce your sugar cravings?

- Are you enjoying weekly trips to the farmers' market (if there's one in your area), where you can buy quality, organic or noncertified organic veggies, fruits, and meats?

- Are you buying fewer foodstuffs from cans, jars, or packages and more real, alive, nutrient-rich foods?

- Have you experimented with the nutritional powerhouses flax seeds, chia seeds, and cacao?

- Are you now choosing low-glycemic fruit for dessert, especially after dinner?

- Are you drinking half your weight in ounces of water throughout the day?

- Have you begun to let go of processed, white carbs and experiment with whole grains such as quinoa or brown rice?

- Are you trying the recipes at the back of this book?

- Are you starting to post your sugar-free recipes on my Facebook fan page so others can try them?

If these seem like a lot of changes to make in one week, simply refer back to this chapter as you enter Weeks Five and Six, so that you can keep making positive food changes a regular part of your life.

Now, you're ready to move into Week Five, where you'll focus on ways to train your Mind to help guide you on your Beyond Sugar Shock adventure.

## CHAPTER 9

## WEEK FIVE

# YOUR MIND: CALM YOUR CRAVINGS WITH COOL TOOLS GALORE & BEFRIEND YOUR SWEET IMPERFECT SELF

### Affirmation: Connie's Simple 7 D's always calm my cravings and make them go poof!

Most sugar addicts grapple with the same challenges when it comes to stomping out those seductive carbs and sweets. In fact, one of the biggest questions people ask me when they hear me talk or hire me to coach them is, "*How do I combat my sugar cravings?*"

Help is here! In fact, we'll devote most of this week to helping you calm your cravings.

You see, your urges to splurge aren't just caused by physical reasons. Often, your cravings are driven by a variety of emotional, psychological, and spiritual factors, including not enough sweetness in your life. But you can train your brain to easily dismiss your irrational yearnings.

To save you from your *must-have-sweets-now moments* when your nagging, childlike, temper-tantrum-like voice keeps badgering you for The Sweet White Stuff, you'll discover how to do such simple tactics as My 7 D's, BreathWork (from my friend Dr. Brian Alman); Metta, or Loving-Kindness; Meditation (an ancient Buddhist practice); and other super-simple cravings conquerors. These powerful tools will *quickly* rescue you anytime, anywhere.

In this chapter, you'll also get simple tips to disband your triggers and saboteurs, playfully *Say "No!" with Sass!* to meddling *Sugar Pushers*, and eat mindfully so you can savor the flavors of those alive, quality foods.

Remember, it's natural at times to feel familiar S.A.D. longings. Of course, your mind is just playing games with you. But you're in control.

These are your choices:

**S.A.D.:** That's when you fall for the old diet logic and think, *A few cookies won't make any difference.* (Who hasn't said that?) And, I'm also willing to bet that you've often made the excuse, *I've already blown my diet. Why not just keep going?*

**SWEET:** That's when you kick those pointless, intrusive, negative thoughts to the curb and decide to act on behalf of your highest good and stay on track with quality foods and thinking.

It's your decision.

## Make Peace with Your Cravings

As you learn new ways to release your cravings, the most important thing to remember is that cravings are only temporary. Step outside yourself and regard your cravings as challenges and opportunities to do some inner exploration. All you need to do is pause, watch, and listen carefully to your calm inner voice, not the irrational one that nudges you into self-destructive carb behavior. No matter how far you've strayed into the sugar abyss, you can always course-correct and put yourself on a better, healthier path.

Now, here are this week's steps to counteract any temptations to fall back into your old sugary routines.

### Affirmation: I am the master of my cravings. They're only visiting me to give me valuable information.

Week Five: **YOUR MIND**
**STEP 1:** Curb Your Cravings with Cool Tools
**STEP 2:** Disband Your Triggers and Saboteurs
**STEP 3:** Eat Mindfully, Savor the Flavors, & Find Your True Taste Buds
**STEP 4:** Laugh, Play & Say "No!" with Sass

## STEP 1: CURB YOUR CRAVINGS WITH COOL TOOLS

## Affirmation: I easily ride out my cravings using Connie's 7 D's.

Let's set the scene first. It's a Monday afternoon at the office, about 3:00 P.M., and you've hit a slump. There's a jar of bright, shiny candies on your co-worker's desk. For hours, you've been *so close* to grabbing a handful, especially after your boss said you have to work late. Or maybe it's 8:30 P.M., and you're home waiting for your spouse, who is two hours late. You've been waiting to eat dinner with your honey, and you're starving. You'd love to nosh on those potato chips sitting in the cupboard.

Those first few minutes or seconds when you come face-to-face with your cravings are crucial. You can act impulsively and give yourself immediate satisfaction and what you *think* you want, or you can stop, pause, and reconsider by asking yourself, *What do I really want?*

You'll get several techniques here to calm your cravings. Just find the ones that work for you. Your goal is to build a powerful arsenal of tools on which you can rely whenever you're faced with tough situations.

## My Simple 7 D's

When my book *Sugar Shock!* first came out, I unveiled what were then my 6 D's, which had helped me back in 1998, and which I've refined since then. Readers loved them. My clients now swear by them, too.

But one day during a radio interview, when the fun, affable, open-minded host asked me about this process, I unexpectedly came up with one more D tool, which is now #6. My interviewer cracked up. Since then, this addition has been a huge hit with private clients and members of my Sugar Freedom Now Course. It's now time to invite My Simple 7 D's into your life:

1.  **Delay!** When something sugary calls out to you, first, do what I call *creative procrastination.* Look at a nearby clock, your watch, or cell phone to mark the time. Next, promise yourself that you won't give

in to your cravings for 15 minutes. You just won't do anything. Then, before you take any action, get going in other ways . . .

2. **Distance yourself!** Get away from any and all temptations! If you're anywhere near an ice cream store, supermarket, bakery, or drugstore, make a fast escape. If you happen to have brought home your favorite sweets—not something I recommend—immediately shove them down the garbage chute. Your immediate goal is to create a safe haven where your intense cravings can subside.

3. **Distract!** Use distraction for your highest good. That means do something constructive in those 15 minutes. Call a good friend or a Break-Free Buddy. Organize papers on your desk. Stand up, if you can, and stretch. Do 15 minutes of bursting. Listen and boogie to your favorite Woo-Hoo, Feel-Good Tune. Take a catnap. Do Ho'oponopono. Remember, you have only 15 minutes to fill.

4. **Decode!** Now that you've put some distance between you and your cravings, begin to do Sugary Soul Searching. Ask yourself the 5 W's & 1 H. *Who or what is bothering me? What foods am I craving? When is this happening? Where am I? Why do I want them now? How will I feel later if I cave in to my cravings?*

5. **Decide!** Now, commit to yourself that *this time*, you'll choose in favor of your beautiful body, clever mind, and ever-expanding spirit. Decide that you want a healthier, happier, sexier, fulfilling life *far more* than you want those sweets.

6. **Diss!** Now comes the most fun part. As you probably know, *diss* is slang for disrespect. So what you'll do is diss that tempting junk food. How? You literally stick out your tongue with contempt! Seriously! Of course, if people are around, you can just pretend to do it. Either way, I'm willing to bet you'll smile, or even chuckle.

7. **Delight!** It's now time to rejoice that you've made this awesome decision to conquer that craving. Pat yourself on the back. Revel in relief and self-pride that you proactively got off your must-have-sugar ledge.

If you're still tempted by those chips or candies, simply repeat My Simple 7 D's again. And if you're still irked by sugar cravings—which I doubt you will be—do this powerful process for another 15 minutes.

By the end of one to three rounds of the 7 D's, you'll have gained meaningful perspective on your cravings and gotten involved in a useful project. More important, you'll have gained confidence that you can do this again and again. And those sweets will have lost their appeal.

## Do BreathWork with Weight Loss Expert Dr. Brian Alman

This next powerful cravings-calming tool comes from Brian Alman, Ph.D., author of *Keep it Off* and *The Voice: Overcome Negative Self-Talk and Discover Your Inner Wisdom*.

He calls this technique BreathWork, and he developed it after working with spiritual masters in India. This tactic can help you get through anything, Dr. Alman says, including nighttime cravings, difficult people, self-anger, stress, pain, frustration about your body, relationship concerns, money challenges, and loneliness.

**YOU'RE A HAPPY, SUCCESSFUL SUGAR KICKER WHEN . . .**

Cravings hit you, and you greet them as you would an old friend who just returned from a trip to a foreign land, where she or he discovered valuable insights to share with you.

1. "First, accept your breathing as it is," Dr. Alman explains. "Don't count. Don't even push in or out your diaphragm. After three to four breaths, your breathing will relax. When you accept your breathing as it is, you get a glimpse of how it feels to accept yourself as you are."

2. "Now, on your exhale, say your own name silently to yourself. Keep breathing and saying your name on the exhale until you feel grounded and connected with yourself. Even 30 seconds of this will give you a great benefit."

3. "Finally, on your inhales, silently state your goal—which, in your case, is winning out over your sugar addiction or weight issues. Then, take three to ten breaths like this, all in an accepting way."

"BreathWork can be a powerful technique to conquer your cravings, because by focusing on your breath, you're calming yourself," Dr. Alman explains. "Plus, your focus will shift away from food—and toward your intentions at a deep and cellular level—when you think, breathe, and bridge your goal with your name."

Isn't that a cool technique?

## More Simple Ways to Calm Your Cravings

Here are more powerful ways to quiet your cravings:

- *Never let yourself get too hungry.* When you're famished, you're more likely to give in to cravings, so make sure to start your day with a healthy breakfast, and eat small, frequent, well-balanced meals throughout the day, recommends dietitian Keri Gans, R.D., author of *The Small Change Diet: 10 Steps to a Thinner, Healthier You.*

- *Eat fiber, protein, and fat at meals and snacks.* This helps keep your blood-sugar levels stable by controlling the release of hormones such as insulin and glucagon.

- *Crowd out your cravings.* When you consume healthy, nutrient-dense foods, water, and beverages that are good for you *earlier in the day*, you'll have less room or desire for unhealthy foods. So explains Joshua Rosenthal, founder and director of the Institute for Integrative Nutrition.

- *Cut back on coffee.* When you have coffee along with sugar (the coffee-and-donut effect), you could trigger a roller-coaster ride of high blood-sugar levels, which can lead to low blood sugar and cravings.

- *Drink one or two glasses of water.* Your desire for sweets in the evening may be a signal that you need water. A glass or two of water may be all you need for your cravings to subside.

- *Cut down on salt.* The next time you crave sweets, just ask yourself if you've been eating too much salt, suggests diet expert Dr. Ann Louise Gittleman.

- *Trick your taste buds with something sour.* Jonny Bowden, C.N., C.N.S., Ph.D., author of *The Most Effective Natural Cures on Earth*, recommends that when you get sugar cravings, try a sour pickle or a hot pepper instead. In other words, pick a food from a different taste family.

- *Do "urge surfing."* Just ride out your craving like you're riding a wave on a surfboard, recommended the now-late psychology professor G. Alan Marlatt, Ph.D., and author of *Relapse Prevention*. As my coaching clients have found, usually, within 15 to 30 minutes, your cravings build, crest, break, and then subside—*if* you don't act on them.

- *Brush your teeth.* The small amount of sugar in your toothpaste (if it has any) may be just enough to satisfy your craving, says Dr. Nancy Appleton.

- *Inhale away your cravings.* Smell pleasurable, aromatic essential oils such as lavender, jasmine, vanilla, or rose. Or try fruity scents such as orange, lemon, or tangerine. (Learn more about scents in the Remarkable Resources section at the back of the book.)

- *Pamper yourself.* Find out if you really want sugar or just to feel loved and appreciated.

- *Cuddle and cradle your cravings like a mother calming her fussy baby.* Because your craving is like a screaming tot trying to get attention, listen to it and acknowledge it without judgment, blame, guilt, or criticism, suggests Lilian Cheung, D.Sc., R.D., co-author of *Savor: Mindful Eating, Mindful Life* with Vietnamese Buddhist Zen master Thich Nhat Hanh. When you do this, the craving loses its strength, and you'll calm down, she says. Then, you can find out why your craving hit in the first place.

### Adventurcise: My Favorite Cravings-Calming Techniques

The next time I get a craving, I'll use these techniques.

1. _____

2. _____

3. _____

You're now ready to go out there and succeed no matter what temptations come your way. I crown you a Successful Cravings-Conqueror!

*"Stressed spelled backwards is desserts. Coincidence? I think not!"*

— AUTHOR UNKNOWN

## STEP 2: DISBAND YOUR TRIGGERS AND SABOTEURS

## Affirmation: I easily recognize my top triggers and saboteurs so they lose their power over me.

Although cutting back on sugar consumption is rapidly gaining momentum across the country and the world, most people around you will still be indulging in—or overdosing on—pies, pasta, potato chips, and more. And, of course, you'll also be surrounded by droves of fast-food places, ice cream shops, and bakeries.

Your goal then is to be on the lookout for situations or people who may threaten your new sugar-free life. In other words, it's time to disband your triggers and saboteurs. Once you're prepared for these undesired or unexpected events or circumstances, you can defuse their power or simply avoid them altogether.

## Beware of Tricky Triggers

First, let's look at how you can avoid threatening triggers. For instance:

- *Sugar Challenge:* You see stacks of candy bars while waiting in line to buy toilet paper at the drugstore. Remember, they're laid out in such a way to entice you and get you to buy them. *Solution:* Give your attention instead to intriguing magazine covers.

- *Sugar Challenge:* You pass by a donut place or café where the aroma is alluring. *Solution:* Go find (or buy yourself) some flowers and smell them instead.

- *Sugar Challenge:* You're really tired. That's a big trigger for many. *Solution:* Take a nap, boogie to your Woo-Hoo, Feel-Good Tune, call a Break-Free Buddy, or listen to a ten-minute meditation download (get one for free at www.BeyondSugarShock.com).

- *Sugar Challenge:* You're at a party where many desserts or culprit carbs are offered. *Solution:* Focus instead on the fascinating guests and fill up on bulky vegetables and quality protein sources.

- *Sugar Challenge:* It's that time of month again, and you're at the mercy of your hormones. *Solution:* Remember my tip to freeze fruits and have them for dessert? Grab a handful of frozen blueberries and enjoy!

- *Sugar Challenge:* You're stressed out, sad, lonely, frustrated, depressed, or dissatisfied with your significant other. *Solution:* Start doing My Simple 7 D's, BreathWork, or listen to your Woo-Hoo, Feel-Good Tune.

Now examine your triggers.

## Adventurcise: My Biggest Triggers

These are my most common triggers. What can I do to avoid them?

1. _____

2. _____

3. _____

4. _____

5. _____

## Watch Out for Well-Intentioned Saboteurs and Sugar Pushers

**YOU'RE A HAPPY, SUCCESSFUL SUGAR KICKER WHEN . . .**
You find new, spiritual, health-minded friends and stay away from your former sugar cronies.

The dilemma with saboteurs is that they often appear trustworthy, loyal, and helpful. It's also important to bear in mind that there's a good chance they're hooked on sweets themselves, which may be why they dismiss your sugar-free ways as extreme or unnecessary. Remember, you and I used to be in their shoes, so don't hold their sugar attachment against them. But be prepared for resistance. In fact, don't be surprised if some people roll their eyes or look at you askance upon hearing that you're skipping sweets.

These *Sugar Pushers*—as I call them in fun and jest—pop up almost everywhere. You'll find them at holiday get-togethers with the family, at the office, and at children's birthday parties.

Now, to be fair, most saboteurs don't intend to interfere with your goals. They probably buy into the sugar-is-love theory, and like most people, they want you to join them in bonding over sugary junk. Or perhaps they don't want to look at their own sugar issues.

Some saboteurs to watch out for include:

- Co-workers who keep jars of candies and stacks of cookies at their desks.

- Busybodies. You know, the people who nag you and say, *"A little piece of cake won't hurt."*

- Friends, friends of friends, or well-intentioned relatives, who, in their efforts to be the best possible hosts, keep offering you sweets. Until you feel secure enough to turn down desserts, you may want to stay away from these events. If you still want to get together with these folks, it's easiest to pick a non-food-related environment such as a park, museum, or gym. You also can plan an appointment immediately afterward so you have to dash out early.

- Your former ice-cream-and-cookies-eating buddies. You may have to avoid your former sugar cronies the way recovering alcoholics often shun their previous drinking buddies.

Now, do some careful planning. Soon you'll be ready to tackle almost any situation.

## Adventurcise: My Biggest Saboteurs

I plan to watch out for the following saboteurs. What can I do to avoid them?

1. _____

2. _____

3. _____

4. _____

5. _____

You'll want to revisit this Adventurcise again, whenever you feel certain functions or people are encouraging you to abandon your new, healthy, sugar-free plan.

## STEP 3: EAT MINDFULLY, SAVOR THE FLAVORS & FIND YOUR TRUE TASTE BUDS

### Affirmation: I take time to savor the flavors and textures of every bite I eat.

If you're like most people hooked on quickie carbs, you numb out and become mindless about your eating experience. I'm going to teach you to eat mindfully so you can not only learn to savor the flavors but also get back in touch with what I call your *true taste buds*.

Mindful eating helps you become more aware of just how hungry you are, how quickly you eat, what foods you choose, and how much you consume. It also helps you enjoy your food and not overeat, according to clinical psychologist Jean Kristeller, Ph.D., an Indiana State University psychology professor emeritus, who developed a mindfulness-eating meditation program to help people with binge eating disorder gain control and shed weight.

Meditation also helps you shift your relationship to eating and food so you can experience what Dr. Kristeller describes as "a feeling of joyful awareness without struggle. You come from a place of acceptance and curiosity, and you experience the flavor of foods in a different way."

Meditating, as you learned earlier, brings many benefits, including reducing stress. It also can help you to cut back on culprit carbs. In fact, meditators don't feel compelled to "chase the flavor," and they're "satisfied with one or two fully conscious bites of a favorite food," Dr. Kristeller says.

With mindful eating, "you want to engage all six senses, beyond just taste," explains Lilian Cheung, D.Sc., R.D. In other words, you'll appreciate your food more by tasting, as well as seeing, smelling, touching, hearing, and thinking about it. As a mindful eater, you also want to honor your food, eat in modest portions, chew thoroughly, and savor the flavors, Cheung suggests.

## Adventurcise: How to Eat Mindfully with Dr. Jean Kristeller

This eating Adventurcise, courtesy of Dr. Kristeller, will help you determine how hungry you really are and develop *gourmet* versus *gluttonous* habits.

- First, select a location where you can sit comfortably.

- Now, pick a food. You might want to use one raisin or one almond. Yes, just one.

- Put it on a plate or napkin in front of you.

- Sit upright, with your feet on the floor, and become quiet.

- If you're comfortable closing your eyes, do that. If not, gaze at a spot in front of you.

- Bring your awareness to your breath. Take two or three deeper breaths.

- Open your eyes. Pick up the raisin or nut.

- Examine it, smell it, and put it in your mouth. Explore its taste and feel.

- Notice your thoughts, feelings, or associations.

- Finally, chew it slowly and explore its tastes and textures. Chew as long as you need to so you fully savor the experience.

- When you're ready, swallow it.

- Notice what it feels like to bring the food into your body.

- Observe any anxieties, questions, or judgments that may arise.

- As you finish, focus again on your breath and body.

- Appreciate that you're alive because of the energy you receive from food, which is made possible thanks to people around the world.

# DANA KENNEDY

### "How I Went a Year Without Candy"

*Note from Connie: Can you quit your favorite candies, cookies, cakes, ice cream, pastries, and sugar-based desserts for 365 days and chronicle your candy-curbing adventures publicly, with panache, humor, and literary aplomb? That's what talented journalist Dana Kennedy—who contributes to AOL News, and* People *and* Time *magazines—did on her entertaining, insightful, healthily addictive A Year Without Candy blog, www.AYearWithoutCandy.com, from Feb. 28, 2010, to Feb. 28, 2011.*

**On Unsuccessfully Trying to Kick Before:** "I've tried to quit candies and sweets so many times before, and I'd last anywhere from four days to two weeks. I'd always lose my motivation and find some reason to go back to sugar even though I knew there's no upside to it; I got stuck in a cycle of being discouraged that I couldn't get the monkey off my back."

**The Blog Kept Me Accountable:** "Unwittingly, I did the perfect thing for my personality, which was to issue a public challenge to myself. The blog was like my conscience. People could tell me all day long how bad candy is for me, what emotional effects it has on me, and what [nutrient-poor] ingredients are in it, but what gave me more motivation was being accountable to somebody or something. And in my mind, I had millions of readers who were just waiting for me to fail, and I couldn't do that. It would be a total defeat and humiliation."

**How I've Changed:** "I haven't had some miraculous Tony-Robbins-meets-Oprah-Winfrey insta-changes. But I feel happier, my skin looks better, emotionally I am calmer, and it's easier to get along with people. Plus, giving up candy and sugar-based desserts has given me more energy than ever. And after resolving some thyroid issues, I finally lost 13 pounds."

**Getting Support from Unexpected Places:** "What's been really surprising is the number of people who have reacted positively and wrote to say that they were inspired and have been helped by things they've learned on the blog. It's a completely different experience [to quit sugar while writing a blog] than to kick sweets [by myself]."

**My Slips Taught Me to Watch It:** "I've had a few relapses like some rice pudding three nights in a row after an appendectomy. But I wrote about it, and then I stopped. What my slips showed me is how easy it would be for me to go right back to the way I was. It's going to be up to me to manage [my sugar addiction] for the rest of my life."

**On Staying off Sugar in the Future:** "I don't know what the future holds, but I've realized that I've had enough sugar to last a lifetime. Quitting candies and other sweets hasn't been anywhere near as much of a struggle as I thought it would. But I'm still being vigilant [even though] I've gotten used to not eating candy, and it's not too much of a struggle to stick with the plan."

## Blog or Journal About Your Sugar-Free Adventures

You're already keeping track of what you eat and how much you exercise in a food diary. Like Dana, you may also benefit by putting your feelings, frustrations, thoughts, dreams, and worries into words. Journaling is a powerful transformational tool that can bring you closer to your true self, give you *Aha!* Insights, and put desired distance between you and your sugar habit.

You also might want to go public by starting a blog to share your challenges or successes with readers. These days, more and more sugar-free bloggers or weight-loss bloggers are gathering supportive, encouraging fans while they help themselves out.

Get links to dozens of sugar-free or weight-loss blogs at *my* blog, www .SugarShockBlog.com.

## Tips to Blog While Quitting Sugar or Releasing Weight from Journalist Dana Kennedy

Here are some tips from Kennedy on how to make blogging work for you.

**How to Begin:** "Do what I did. Somehow make it a challenge to yourself."

**You Don't Have to Publicize It:** "First, you can control who sees it. You don't have to tell anyone that the blog even exists. You can do the blog for yourself and use an obscure domain name. But don't put anything in it that you don't want the world to see."

**Blogging Doesn't Always Mean Writing:** "If you're more visually oriented, do a video. I think it'd be hilarious to go to your favorite bakery and shoot what candy bars you wish you could have today! Or you could take a photo, which is worth, as they say, 1,000 words, and just write one line of text. You can do anything. "

STEP 4: LAUGH, PLAY & SAY "NO!" WITH SASS

## Affirmation: I now laugh, chuckle, and giggle more than ever before!

Now, your goal is to consciously begin chuckling, giggling, laughing, and lightening up on a daily basis. Why not regard your former habit with a little levity? You'll find that it's easier and more life affirming to take this approach.

For centuries, philosophers, scholars, physicians, and scientists have talked about humor's therapeutic value. Even the Bible attests to the importance of a "merry heart." The late Norman Cousins, a former *Saturday Review* editor, was among the first to suggest that laughter can heal you. He made a point to watch Marx Brothers movies and *Candid Camera* reruns. What happened next is amazing: he went into remission from *ankylosing spondylitis*, a debilitating rare disease of the connective tissues.

Ultimately, Cousins' adventure into laughter became big news, resulting in a 1976 article in *The New England Journal of Medicine* and leading to his groundbreaking book, *Anatomy of an Illness as Perceived by the Patient*.

Ever since the magazine editor's experiment with humor and healing, many people have put a laughter plan into place when facing a serious illness or challenge. That's why you now want to use humor to help heal you, too.

### It's Healthy to Laugh

Laughter is now universally regarded as good medicine. Studies even demonstrate that the body's major physiologic systems are stimulated during mirthful laughter. Here are some of laughter's benefits:

- Laughter can improve vascular (related to blood vessels) function, according to a study in the *American Journal of Cardiology,* which also showed that watching a documentary instead of a comedy didn't provide this benefit.

- Repetitive "mirthful laughter"—or what researchers call *Laughercise*— causes the body to respond in a way that's similar to moderate physical exercise, according to scientists from Loma Linda University's School of Allied Health Professions. After watching humorous videos, subjects also experienced improvements in mood, immune activity, cholesterol, and blood pressure.

• Laughter has a variety of physiological, psychological, social, spiritual, and quality-of-life benefits, including muscle relaxation and a reduction in cortisol (a hormone released in response to stress), according to more research from the Organización Mundial de la Risa in Barcelona, Spain.

You get the idea. It's time to laugh.

*"Laughter is the most inexpensive and most effective wonder drug. Laughter is a universal medicine."*

— NOBEL PRIZE WINNER BERTRAND RUSSELL

## Go Ahead: Laugh at Your Old Sugar Habit and You "On" Sugar

Ultimately, your goal is to find humor in your addiction. When you laugh at something—even something painful like your sugar habit—you strip away its power over you and gain control over it.

To get those belly laughs started, try some or all of the following:

• Read funny books or listen to audio programs from such humorists, TV personalities, or authors as Jon Stewart, David Sedaris, Dave Barry, or Bill Cosby. Spend time at a library, bookstore, or on the Internet to find books or movies that tickle your funny bone.

• Watch your favorite sitcoms, sketch comedy shows such as *Saturday Night Live,* or cute animal videos on YouTube.

• Rent or buy movies with funny comedians such as Chris Rock, Robin Williams, Whoopi Goldberg, Jim Carrey, Woody Allen, Steve Martin, Adam Sandler, or Mel Brooks.

• Go to a comedy club, take an improv class, or show up at an open-mike program. (All three of these are a blast, as I can attest.)

• Go ahead and make fun of yourself and your sugar addiction in front of friends or family members.

## Playcise: My Silly-on-Sugar Behavior

See the humor in outrageous things you've done after eating sugar.

On each line, list an unbelievable sugar-inspired action and then what you ate that brought it about.

1._____

2._____

3._____

Thoughts/Conclusions:

_____

_____

## Playcise: Give Your Sugar Creature a Silly Name

Now, you'll undertake another fun Playcise. Give a silly name to your sugar-induced, Jekyll-and-Hyde-like alter ego.

Go ahead and call yourself a Sugar Bitch or Sugar Demon, if you like! By the way, over the years, I've gotten lots of laughter mileage by calling myself an *Ex-Sugar Shrew*. Labeling this creature puts a huge distance between her and me, and lets me step outside myself and easily break away from that former, unsavory critter. It's now your turn.

Here are some wacko names for the creature I became. What was I eating then?

1._____

2._____

3._____

Thoughts/Conclusions:

_____

_____

169

## Adventurcise: Laughter Planning

Here are three funny books that I could buy or check out from the library:

1. _____

2. _____

3. _____

Here are three TV sitcoms I could watch:

1. _____

2. _____

3. _____

Here are three funny movies I could rent:

1. _____

2. _____

3. _____

Here are three things to do that would definitely make me laugh!

1. _____

2. _____

3. _____

**Affirmation: I'm having so much fun standing up
for myself and Saying "No!" with Sass! to sweets.**

## Defuse Dessert Tension with Humor: Say "No!" with Sass!

For years, I've been bombarded with requests from private coaching clients and participants of my Sugar Freedom Now Course (Break Free of Your Sugar Addiction in 6 Weeks Program) for effective ways to say no when well-meaning Sugar Pushers keep trying to shove desserts their way.

Get ready now to learn fun ways to Say "No!" with Sass!

When you turn down sugar purveyors, you don't need to give long explanations. Instead, banish awkwardness with cheerful, good-natured remarks, jovial bantering, and comedic quips. Try a big smile, a wink, a chuckle, a laugh, a mischievous look, or even a flirtatious flick of your head (if appropriate).

What's more, when you Say "No!" with Sass!, it underscores the idea that going sugar-free is fun. Here are some ideas on how to playfully reply:

- *No thanks—I'm sweet enough!*

- *No can do. Just think of me as Superman. Sugar is my kryptonite.*

- *Thank you, no. Sugar used to be the love of my life. But we've had a nasty breakup. I won't ever take him (or her) back.*

- *Dessert? No thanks, I'm the designated driver.*

- *I'd love to, but my sweet tooth has a habit of turning into fangs.*

- *No dessert for me. I knew I had a sugar problem when I listed Sara Lee and Ben & Jerry as job references, and my physician as Dr Pepper.*

Now have fun coming up with your own quips.

## Playcise: My Five Favorite Ways to Say "No!" with Sass!

What are your favorite sassy lines?

1. _____

2. _____

3. _____

4. _____

5. _____

For more ideas on how to Say "No!" with Sass!, visit my Sugar Shock Blog or Beyond Sugar Shock website.

## Your Mind Is Now Enrolled in Releasing the Sugar

This week, you made some powerful strides. First, you learned how to get your mind engaged by learning a variety of cutting-edge, acclaimed techniques to curb your cravings. From there, you discovered how to identify those people and places that can thwart your success. You also learned how to become a more mindful, conscious eater. And you finally took a playful, humorous approach to life and your sugar habit. You even discovered how to fight off those annoying Sugar Pushers with grace, charm, and dignity (and a little sass). Now it's time for a quick review.

## Before You Head into Week Six, Are You Using Simple Cravings-Stopping Tools to Stay on Track?

- When tempted, are you using My Simple 7 D's? How have they helped you?

- Are you now observing and also welcoming your cravings, because they provide valuable information?

- Have you tried such powerful cravings-calming techniques as BreathWork?

- Have you identified your biggest sugar triggers and figured out how to deal with them?

- Have you decided whether to totally avoid your top saboteurs or do different things with them such as meeting at the gym or going for a walk?

- Are you now eating more mindfully and savoring your meals as never before?

- Have you found favorite movies, TV shows, books, and other activities that make you laugh? What are they?

- Are you seeing the humor in your former S.A.D. ways?

- Have you come up with your own ways to Say "No!" with Sass? Have you shared them with us on my Facebook fan page?

Hurrah! You're now ready to move on to the final week of your Beyond Sugar Shock adventure.

## CHAPTER 10

## WEEK SIX

# YOUR SPIRIT: JOYOUSLY, EASILY, EFFORTLESSLY RELEASE YOUR ADDICTION AND GLIDE INTO SUGAR FREEDOM

**Affirmation: I'm now joyously gliding into Sugar Freedom! Woo-Hoo!**

Congratulations! You've now reached the final week of *Beyond Sugar Shock*! I hope that you've found this to be a thrilling, nourishing, soul-nurturing journey, and your life has been opening up and expanding in many wonderful, powerful ways.

During our past five weeks together, you've been building a sturdy, unshakable platform to make powerful, positive changes. Now, I invite you to take a few minutes to go back and review the healthier, harmonious habits you've been adopting. Take a fresh look at the many easy tools and practices you've learned to soothe yourself—especially ones you may have overlooked or dismissed.

Please reconsider them as you build your toolbox of powerful techniques that easily catapult you into the amazing next phase of your life, in which you enjoy the glorious bounty of fresh, real, nourishing foods, people, and activities. With a little more time and practice, your smart, simple tactics will become nearly automatic to you, and you'll get even faster, longer-lasting results.

It's time to address your Spirit again. To begin, you'll learn to treat yourself often with what I call *Sweet Relief Goodies*, which you can consistently lean on for true comfort instead of using and abusing S.A.D. so-called comfort foods. You'll get solace by moving in joyous, sexy, raucous, sensuous ways that ignite every cell in your body and take you to a peaceful, calming, joyful, spiritual place.

Next, you'll learn about how to give yourself self-compassion if you slip and fall off the no-sugar wagon. I don't expect you to be perfect—nor should you. Learning to be nurturing and self-compassionate will allow you to be *perfectly imperfect* and still love and approve of yourself.

From there, you'll find interests and hobbies that fascinate and intrigue you and also boost your spirituality. Finally, you'll rest, recharge your batteries, do enriching activities, and hang out with loved ones and friends.

Are you ready for liftoff? Let's go.

Week Six: **YOUR SPIRIT**
**STEP 1:** Treat Yourself with Sweet Relief Goodies like Zumba and Nia
**STEP 2:** Give Yourself Compassion & Be Gentle If You Slip
**STEP 3:** Pursue Your Passions to Get Your Fill Now
**STEP 4:** Savor the Sweetness of Doing Nothing

## STEP 1: TREAT YOURSELF WITH SWEET RELIEF GOODIES LIKE ZUMBA AND NIA

### Affirmation: I now treat myself often and find sweet relief by taking fun fitness classes.

To begin this final powerful week devoted to your Spirit, you'll want to find at least two remarkable physical activities that charge you up; make you feel sexy, confident, courageous, enthusiastic, exhilarated, and spiritual; improve your health and moods; get your mind *off* sugar and quickie carbs; and motivate you so you leave the class or workout determined and ready to succeed. To make this simple for you, I'm sharing with you some of my favorite dance or fitness routines, practices, and classes.

## Join a Zumba Fitness Party

Get ready for fitness fun now. First find an exhilarating, easy-to-follow Zumba Fitness class in your area. These high-energy, downright exciting workouts—which fuse hypnotic Latin rhythms, international music, and simple cardio moves (no complicated choreography to remember)—are easy to find. With a whopping *10 million-plus fans worldwide*, you can get moving at more than 90,000 locations in 110 countries, including hundreds of health clubs, such as Equinox Fitness, Bally Total Fitness Clubs, Curves, Gold's Gym, YMCAs, and Crunch.

Zumba Fitness was created by Colombia-born aerobics instructor and choreographer Alberto Perez when he simply forgot to bring his aerobics music to class one day. "The only option I had was to play music I had in my bag—Latina, salsa, merengue, cumbia, reggaeton, rock 'n' roll, cha-cha, samba, and flamenco—and improvise for one hour," Perez recalls, speaking on my *Gab with the Gurus Radio Show,* before a Zumbathon benefiting the American Heart Association.

Soon, Zumba experienced a meteoric rise in popularity. Why? "It's for every-body—for regular people like you: mothers, executives, lawyers, students. And it's so easy," Perez replies. "It's a party, and people love to party. People don't have time to exercise, but people have time to party. That's why we deliver a party experience."

At the same time, people are building muscles and burning calories (about 500 to 800 calories an hour). "Once you try it, you'll be addicted," predicts Perez, author of *Zumba: Ditch the Workout, Join the Party! The Zumba Weight Loss Program.*

## Work Out Your Body, Mind & Spirit with IntenSati

Next, I urge you to try *intenSati,* a revolutionary, upbeat Mind-Body-Spirit workout that fuses high-energy aerobics, martial arts, dance, and yoga with affirmations to awaken your potential. Created in 2003 by pioneering fitness trainer and motivational speaker Patricia Moreno, the name *intenSati* was created using the words *intention* and *Sati,* a Pali word meaning *mindfulness.* The innovative practice meshes Moreno's passion for fitness with spirituality, optimistic thinking, and meditation.

While you break a sweat, intenSati also teaches you to be more mindful about the words you choose. Not only are you making your body stronger, but you're using affirmations and making yourself feel stronger spiritually and emotionally.

# RICHARD MARTINEZ

## "How 75 Pounds Fell Off & My Confidence Soared"

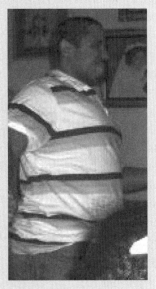

*Note from Connie: When I heard the remarkable story of Richard Martinez (http://22050.zumba.com), one my favorite Zumba Fitness instructors, I just had to share it with you.*

**I'd Been Obese All My Life:** "I grew up eating a lot of traditional Puerto Rican foods—rice and beans, fried pork chops, fried plantains, and refried beans. Everything that could be bad for you, we ate. My parents were never big on vegetables, and my mother fried everything. The more grease, the better. To make matters worse, I was raised in the Bronx, where playing outside wasn't always safe. I was fairly sedentary until age 39. At my heaviest, I reached 260 pounds, and I'm only 5'3"."

**My Turning Point:** "One night, at 2 in the morning, I was sitting in front of the TV, pigging out and wondering how to tackle my weight problem. I'd already tried every fad diet that existed. While channel surfing, I caught a Zumba Fitness infomercial. I figured I had nothing to lose so I ordered the DVDs. When they arrived, I immediately fell in love with the music."

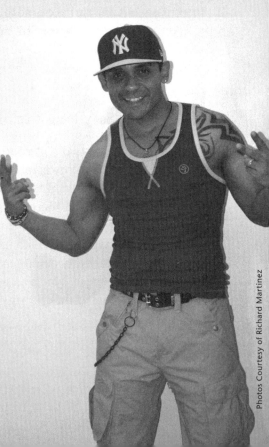

**I Got Hooked on Zumba:** "Then, I took a Zumba Fitness class at the local YMCA and got hooked. There's nothing like the experience of a live class. Everyone is having fun, forgetting their weight problems, enjoying the music and the [simple] choreography, and getting a workout. Zumba is for everyone—regardless of your weight, age, gender, and ethnicity. It's even great for people who are too intimidated to go to a gym."

**Zumba Got Me into Working Out More:** "I never liked working out, but taking Zumba classes got me into the gym, kept me focused and coming back, and inspired me to do other things like body-sculpting, kickboxing, Pilates, running on the treadmill, and swimming. Taking all those classes and eating right allowed me to lose 75 pounds in four and a half months."

Photos Courtesy of Richard Martinez

## Learn Masala Bhangra

Another fun way to move and lift your spirits is with the Masala Bhangra workout, a high-energy, easy-to-follow, cardiovascular and strength-training dance routine that was developed by fitness veteran and choreographer Sarina Jain. She created the name by combining the Hindi word for *spicy* (Masala) with the name of a traditional folk dance from the northern state of Punjab, India (Bhangra).

The Masala Bhangra workout incorporates sensuous, vigorous movements and elements of *Bollywood* (popular Hindi-language films). Essentially, you want to feel like you're at an Indian wedding, explains Jain, who invented this fitness routine in honor of her father, who passed away of cardiac arrest at age 47.

"I want people to walk out of a Masala Bhangra class feeling energized and motivated by the music and dance," says Jain, appearing on my *Gab with the Gurus Radio Show.*

"This is a dance of celebration. That's the type of joy I want to bring to people, where everyone is having so much fun that they don't realize they are getting an awesome cardiovascular and muscle-strengthening workout."

## Celebrate Your Body, Mind, and Spirit with Nia

You also can appreciate the joy of moving by learning Nia, a sensory-based practice that draws on martial arts, dance arts, and healing arts. Designed for all fitness levels, Nia was founded in the early 1980s by Debbie Rosas and Carlos AyaRosas, and it now has some 125,000 fans worldwide, many of whom are weight-loss or health success stories.

It isn't just exercise. "Nia teaches you how to move with the design of your body, listen to what it needs, and live in it in a passionate and joyful way," explains Nia Black Belt teacher and trainer Caroline Kohles, who is also senior director of Health and Wellness at the JCC (Jewish Community Center) in New York City.

## Give These Physical Sweet Relief Goodies Top Priority

I simply cannot stress enough how important it is for you to find fun ways to move your luscious, succulent, sexy behind and body and elevate your Spirit at the same time. To learn more about Zumba, intenSati, Masala Bhangra, and Nia, visit my blog, www.SugarShockBlog.com, and click the Sweet Relief Goodies tab.

Even if right now you feel like a pile of blubber, you'll feel totally different about your figure as soon as you get moving. After at least one of these classes, I predict, you'll leave feeling bright-eyed, animated, joyous, and enraptured.

If these activities aren't your cup of tea, then try bicycling, belly dancing, or find some other activity that you love. And tell us about it, too, on my Facebook fan page and in our SparkTeam.

Ultimately, your goal is to find many favorite Sweet Relief Goodies to lift your spirits over and over, time and time again.

## STEP 2: GIVE YOURSELF COMPASSION & BE GENTLE IF YOU SLIP

## Affirmation: I give myself compassion no matter what.

Many Sugar Kickers—once they've made a decision to let go of their habit—expect themselves to be absolutely perfect 100 percent of the time. Of course, perfectionism is impossible. So now, please cut yourself some slack. No matter how well you follow *Beyond Sugar Shock*, you want to be gentle, loving, and completely accepting of yourself.

Indeed, as a delightfully imperfect human being, you may "slip" at some point on your healthy adventure. And that's just fine. It's even to be expected.

But it's how you treat yourself *immediately after* you slip that can make or break your mood, make numbers on your scale go up or down, and bring about or rob you of peace of mind.

So if you do slip, be very gentle with yourself. "When you have self-compassion and treat yourself with care and concern—like a friend or loved one—you're more apt to eat [only] when you're hungry, stop when you're full, rest when you're tired, and move when you feel energized. By doing that, you will lose weight naturally," says psychotherapist Jean Fain, L.I.C.S.W., M.S.W., author of *The Self-Compassion Diet*.

A growing body of research now reveals that self-compassion is *exactly* what you need when embarking on a diet or meal plan—and especially if you slip. Just review startling results from a landmark Wake Forest University study which was designed to promote self-compassion among so-called restrictive eaters (dieters) and guilty eaters (those who "blew" their diets).

First, researchers instructed 84 female undergraduate students—31 percent of whom already were on a diet—to eat a "forbidden food," a donut, in this case. Half the participants were taught in advance how to give themselves compassion after partaking in the "no-no" snack. Then, afterward, when offered unwrapped candies, they didn't start to emotionally eat. On the other hand, their self-critical counter-parts—who didn't get a self-compassion lesson in advance—ate a lot more of the "no-no" candies when they were offered.

In other words, the researchers found that self-compassion seems to be an *antidote* to the self-criticism and emotional distress that fuels emotional eating. The research—which was reviewed in an article in the *Journal of Social and Clinical Psychology*—found that "people who treat themselves with compassion when they overeat might be more successful at regulating their eating . . . "

Self-compassion is so incredibly powerful and important that it can color your entire outlook on life.

"People who are self-compassionate are much less anxious, happier, more optimistic, more satisfied with their lives, and more motivated to grow and change," contends pioneering self-compassion researcher Kristin Neff, Ph.D., author of *Self-Compassion: Stop Beating Yourself Up and Leave Insecurity Behind.*

In fact, the idea that being self-critical is a good motivator is *"an absolute myth,"* asserts Dr. Neff, who is associate professor of human development and culture at the University of Texas at Austin.

"All research shows that if you criticize yourself, you become depressed and stop believing in yourself," Dr. Neff explained during an interview on my *Gab with the Gurus Radio Show.* "The motivational power of self-criticism comes from *fear,* but the motivational power of compassion comes from *love.*"

## Show Self-Compassion by Doing Metta, or Loving-Kindness, Meditation

Self-compassion is so critical to your success that from now on, you want to spend a few minutes every day giving it to yourself.

What you'll do is a simplistic form of the ancient Buddhist Metta, or Loving-Kindness, Meditation, which has soared in popularity in recent years, thanks to such people as meditation master Sharon Salzberg, one of the first to bring this Eastern tradition to the West, beginning with her bestseller, *LovingKindness: The Revolutionary Art of Happiness*.

*Metta* means kindness, friendliness, goodwill, benevolence, fellowship, amity, nonviolence, and a strong wish for the welfare and happiness of others. In other words, it encompasses an attitude of selfless love. To do Metta meditation:

First, focus on yourself by silently repeating these four phrases:

*May I be safe.*
*May I be happy.*
*May I be healthy.*
*May I live with ease.*

Next, extend your loving-kindness to a loved one:

*May you be safe.*
*May you be happy.*
*May you be healthy.*
*May you live with ease.*

Now, think bigger. Envision sending out Metta to your neighbors, anyone with sugar issues, and the entire human race. That's when you say:

*May we be safe.*
*May we be happy.*
*May we be healthy.*
*May we live with ease.*

If you like, you can even shorten these phrases into mantras such as *safe*, *happy*, *healthy*, and *ease*. Or if you'd like to rewrite these phrases, go ahead and take poetic license. Just make your Metta statements meaningful to you.

Or do one of my favorite techniques to boost your mood and morale and calm your anxieties. Look at a photo of yourself as an adorable baby or child and spread warmth to the beautiful person you see. Who doesn't want to share loving-kindness with a cute kid?

Ultimately, this simple tool will help transport you away from your fear and self-loathing and move you into self-love. Now, here's some help in advance if you do slip.

## COACH CONNIE'S SWEET SUCCESS STRATEGY

# How to Comfort Yourself After a Slip

- *Give yourself huge, unconditional dose of tenderness and comfort.* Pretend that you're comforting your adorable kid—your inner child, perhaps—who got a big *boo-boo* from falling off her bike.

- *Hug yourself.* Seriously, tenderly touch yourself! Put your hands on your heart or face, or give yourself another gesture of affection. When you receive loving touches, oxytocin (the feel-good hormone) and other opiates are released, which calm you down and lower your cortisol levels.

- *Accept that everyone makes mistakes.* Messing up is part of the human condition, so focus on what's important, which is to be healthy. Don't dwell on the past.

- *Silently reassure yourself.* Comfort yourself by saying something like, *I'm so sorry that you had such a rough time and slipped, but it's understandable because of . . .* (fill in the blank).

- *Act like a compassionate figure or someone who loves you.* Just treat yourself as if you're a compassionate grandmother, loving relative, or even Buddha. "The Buddha's not going to say, *'You fat, stupid, lazy slob!'*" Dr. Neff asserts. "The Buddha's going to say, *'Listen, I care about you, and I don't want you to keep causing yourself to suffer by eating foods that make you feel so bad.'* A compassionate person wants to alleviate your suffering."

- *Do tapping or EFT.* This can help you understand the reasons behind your slip, and how you can prevent another one. (Listen to a special EFT session on www.BeyondSugarShock.com to help you after a slip.)

- *Play a favorite soothing tune.* Sit back and relax. Or if you feel restless, dance to your Woo-Hoo, Feel-Good Tune or another melody that makes you feel triumphant.

- *Do Ho'oponopono.* Remember, that's when you silently say (while thinking of the Divine), *I'm sorry. Please forgive me. Thank you. I love you.*

## STEP 3: PURSUE YOUR PASSIONS TO GET YOUR FILL NOW

### Affirmation: I have a new passion that thrills and fulfills me.

It's now time to shift your focus onto constructive activities that are healthier and more enjoyable than your old S.A.D. ways. In other words, it's time to find or rediscover passions—unrelated to food—so you can *Get Your Fill Now.* To put it bluntly, no one wants to hang out with people obsessed with quitting sugar or culprit carbs. Boring!

## Find Hobbies That Elevate Dopamine and Serotonin

One of the most important ways to begin flipping the switch from Sugar Misery to Sugar Freedom is to have wonderful diversions. Our brain chemistry is even wired for us to create new hobbies, according to neuroscientist David W. Self, Ph.D., professor of psychiatry at the University of Texas, Southwestern Medical Center at Dallas.

"If you stick with a new behavior and repeatedly link it to a reward, which elevates [the neurotransmitters] dopamine and serotonin, the behavior will become more automatic and habitual, and you'll find yourself doing it without giving it much thought," Dr. Self explains.

Your goal, then, is to have things in your life that are far more fun and rewarding than an unhealthy habit that eroded away at the structure of your life.

Psychologist Howard J. Shaffer, Ph.D., C.A.S., director of Harvard Medical School's Division on Addictions, also stresses the importance of doing things that make you happy such as learning new skills, exercising, and finding better substitutes. "Those are the best protections against addictions and best activities to recover from them," he says.

When you make life worth living, you reduce addiction—whether it's to sugar, cocaine, heroin, or something else, explains Dr. Shaffer, who has spent three decades studying and treating addictions. In fact, the people most successful at conquering their addictions are those who recognize that they can make constructive choices, he adds.

## Discover Healthier Passions

Whenever new coaching clients begin working with me, they're often irrationally obsessed with their favorite sweets or culprit carbs. However, soon after we begin, they become wildly passionate about non-food-related activities, such as going on long bicycle rides, taking various gym classes, having more fun with their children, super-charging their marriage or love life, building a business, or rediscovering a hobby that was abandoned years ago.

That's a large part of why I love helping sugar and carb addicts so much. It's utterly thrilling and exhilarating to watch their dramatic transformations.

Your assignment now is to find some things that truly excite you, charge you up, make you burst out into a huge grin and go *Aaaah*, and thrill you in a way that sugar *never ever* can.

People turn to activities that don't serve them, such as bingeing on sugar, because they're unfulfilled, explains Janet Atwood, co-author of *The New York Times* bestseller *The Passion Test: The Effortless Path to Discovering Your Life Purpose.*

"But when you pursue your passions, all of a sudden it becomes easier to stop doing these things because you have a bigger 'Why,'" explains Atwood, speaking on my *Gab with the Gurus Radio Show.*

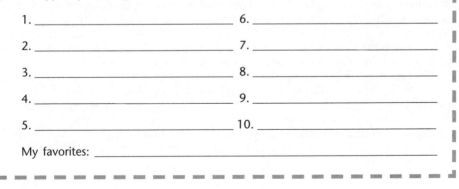

## Playcise: Pick and Pursue Your Passions

It's now time to build your happiness-generating Top 10 Passions List. Start planning playful, laughter-producing, rewarding, mood-lifting activities that can get your mind off the unhealthy Sweet White Stuff and on to sweet pursuits. Make sure to write down activities that you'd like to do, but haven't had time to undertake. And make sure to pick passions that have absolutely nothing to do with sweets.

## My Top 10 Passions List Playcise—Healthy Things I Love to Do

Copy your list onto a three-by-five card to bring with you wherever you go. Also post a copy on your fridge and include another in or near your calendar.

1. _____     6. _____

2. _____     7. _____

3. _____     8. _____

4. _____     9. _____

5. _____     10. _____

My favorites: _____

# MICHELE M.

## SWEET SUCCESS STORY

### "How I Quit Sugar & Rediscovered My Marriage and Great Sex with My Husband."

*Note from Connie:* In April 2010, Michele M., of northern California, joined my Break Free of Your Sugar Addiction in 6 Weeks Program (www.BreakFreeWithConnie.com). I invited Michele to share her sugar saga, because much of what she describes may ring true for you. Plus, her story is so motivating. Because she talks about very intimate, sensitive subjects, Michele asked that her identity be kept a secret.

**Before I Quit Sugar, I Was Often Sick & Tired:** "My blood pressure was so high that my doctor said I might have a stroke. I couldn't breathe right, and I had scary heart palpitations. By 3 P.M. every day, I was exhausted and cranky. I also was overweight—I weighed 143 pounds, but I'm only 5'2". Plus, my intimate relationship with my husband was nonexistent—*I had absolutely no sex drive.*"

**I Hid My Sugar Addiction Like a Drug Addict or Alcoholic:** "It wasn't about willpower for me. I was just like an alcoholic or drug addict [with sugar]. And like most addicts, I hid my addiction. I would make up an excuse to go grocery shopping, and I would buy candy and inhale it in the car before coming home. I would even steal my kids' Halloween candy! For years, I was having a *secret affair with sugar.*"

**I Didn't Want to Stop:** "I didn't want to quit sugar, but I also didn't want to feel so horrible anymore. And I didn't want the guilt. *Sugar was my big relationship.* I turned to sugar when I was down and when I was happy. I'd tried to quit sugar so many times that I lost track. I always had the right intentions, but I couldn't do it alone. It was a very tiring way to live."

**Connie's Sad Sugar Story Woke Me Up:** "I related to Connie's story in her book *Sugar Shock!* about how she became cranky, argumentative, and overly emotional with her boyfriend. I read it to my husband, my mom, and my sister, and I e-mailed it to everyone in my family. I believe that God puts people in my life for a reason, and He led me to Connie."

**Why I Was Successful This Time:** "The reason I was successful kicking sugar this time was Connie's wonderful weekly programs, her coaching, and the daily connections [via e-mails or audio messages] for six weeks. But I was also so ready to change my life. My favorite day of the week was Tuesdays at 5 P.M. Pacific time, when the [Break Free Program] calls took place. I loved the group's accountability and the techniques Connie taught us. After doing this program, even though I've had many stressful family situations, I've been able to deal with everything that has come my way in a positive manner."

**I've Never Felt Better:** "My blood pressure went down with zero exercise. (I couldn't exercise for a year due to painful Plantar fasciitis.) I'm now breathing better; I'm not having heart palpitations anymore; I quickly lost 20 pounds; and I'm full of energy. I'm also happy again. I'm smiling and laughing a lot, and I'm fun to be around."

**Sugar No Longer Has a Hold on Me:** "My cravings have disappeared. And I'm enjoying the natural sweet taste of healthy foods. I even brought my children along for the ride. Living sugar-free is great!"

**My Sex Drive Soared When I Quit Sugar!:** "One of the most exciting things that has happened since I got off sugar is that *my desire for intimacy and love in my marriage is alive and kicking!* Unbelievable how sugar sabotaged that! I never would have thought that living sugar-free would change my sex drive, but it did! My husband and I are having a lot of fun now!"

## Adventurcise: Passion Follow-Up

What did you do? _____

How did it feel to engage in these pursuits? _____

Did you have fun? _____

While you were pursuing your passion, did you think about sweets and simple carbs?

Not at all! _____ A little bit _____ A lot _____

What did you learn? _____

What are your exciting passion plans for next week?_____

Write more about this in your journal or blog.

## STEP 4: SAVOR THE SWEETNESS OF DOING NOTHING

### Affirmation: Today and every day, I take time to Savor the Sweetness of Doing Nothing.

As *Beyond Sugar Shock* winds down, take time off to simply Savor the Sweetness of Doing Nothing. In other words, chill out, unwind, and enjoy yourself. This concept comes from the Italian phrase, *il dolce far niente* ("sweet doing nothing"), which was popularized in Elizabeth Gilbert's best-selling memoir, *Eat, Pray, Love.*

*Il dolce far niente* means hanging out in a café talking with friends, enjoying a leisurely bite to eat, getting engaged in animated conversation, or watching people go by. It's about relishing the pleasure of relaxation and carefree idleness.

The Sweetness of Doing Nothing is completely different from lolling about or wasting time. You're doing nothing *on purpose*.

This is about giving to yourself *the delicious gift of time* with no goals, no obligations, no deadlines, and absolutely no checking off of things on your to-do list.

Skip e-mail, too. And try to declare a time-out—even if just for an hour or two—on checking your text messages or tweets.

This is your chance to recharge, reconnect, rejuvenate, and remember what matters most to you. *Il dolce far niente* is about enjoying the sweetness of the present moment, with no cares in the world.

Your goal is to achieve peace of mind, serenity, and complete relaxation. In our hyper-connected, 24/7 world, you may have to *work* at doing nothing. So here are some tips to get into a Sweetness of Doing Nothing mood:

- *Mark your calendar.* Pick a full day to Savor the Sweetness of Doing Nothing.

- *Take a leisurely bike ride.* During your special time, note that we're not talking about getting a rigorous workout. This is not exercise time.

- *Watch a beautiful sunset.* Pay attention to those vivid, soothing colors that paint the sky.

- *Get out in nature.* Follow in the footsteps of Thoreau and appreciate nature but be careful of ticks, which can spread Lyme disease. (Learn about it by reading my stories—just do a Google search for "Connie Bennett and Lyme disease.")

- *Include friends and family* in your Sweetness of Doing Nothing activities. For instance, enjoy laughter-filled, leisurely walks; do crossword puzzles; or sip sugar-free herbal tea together. By sharing these small, tender moments, you'll deepen your relationships.

Savor the Sweetness of Doing Nothing for a few hours at least once every week. Or, take Do Nothing Breaks daily, whenever possible. Take a leisurely nap, chill out with a magazine, or do something fun with the kids. You get the idea. So, what's your plan for *il dolce far niente*?

### Adventurcise: My Sweetness of Doing Nothing Day

How will you celebrate *il dolce far niente*?

1. _____

2. _____

3. _____

What are three things you can do every day to Savor the Sweetness of Doing Nothing?

1. _____

2. _____

3. _____

## The Sweeter, Full-Life Process

### Affirmation: Every day, I fill myself up with non-food-related sweetness.

Now that you're close to finishing *Beyond Sugar Shock*, I'd like to share a fun, simple technique that I created *just for you*. Use this in the morning or whenever you need a boost of encouragement.

This process is especially effective if you want to raid the fridge, or if you feel angry, lonely, or discouraged.

Just as you'd pour gas into your car when it's empty, do the Sweeter, Full-Life Process to help you when you most need emotional nourishment, spiritual sustenance, or inner peace. You can do this anywhere. Just skip the hand or arm gestures if you're among other people. So, let's get going:

- First, take three deep breaths into your diaphragm.

- With determination in your heart, silently say—or loudly pronounce if you're alone, with your arms thrust in the air—*I am free.*

- Now, gently hug yourself. If you can, slightly rock back and forth. Then say, *I am sweet.* (You may want to do this while looking at a photo of yourself as a baby or child.)

- If you can, extend your arms in front of you as if you're serving someone with a delicious platter of healthy food and gently, appreciatively pronounce, *Life is sweet.*

- Next, lovingly touch your stomach and say, *I feel full.*

- Conclude with, *Thank you, God, for this or better.* If you wish, instead of saying the word *God*, substitute *Universe* or *Universal Intelligence*—or whatever word suits you.

## Affirmation: Woo-Hoo! I am free!

### Your Quick "Cheat Sheet" Recap: Take Your Smart M.E.D.S.

Woo-Hoo! Be proud of yourself.

By completing your six-week Beyond Sugar Shock program, you now have an arsenal of many simple, sweet tools to help you become happier, healthier, slimmer, sexier, and spiritually evolved.

As we conclude our time together, let me share a really easy way to remember most of the tactics and tips that you've learned. Ideally, every day, you'll take some of what I call your Smart M.E.D.S. to make your life continuously rewarding and sweeterlicious.

Your Smart M.E.D.S. can save you often. In fact, as you review this list, jot down the items on your Smart M.E.D.S. list on a 3 x 5 note card or type them into your SmartPhone. That way, if sweets call out to you, you can always take out your list and get reminded the many fun, healthy activities you could do instead of caving in to your sugar cravings. Now, here's your list of effective Smart M.E.D.S.

- **M = Meditate** (in short spurts, if need be); **Mindfully Eat; Move to Music;** and **Motivate with the Masters** (reading and listening to your favorite spiritual leaders).

- **E = Exercise** and **Enjoy** your favorite physical activities and passions; **Embrace Your Emotions; Eat Energy Foods** (Mother Nature's Carb Gifts, as well as ample quality sources of protein and fats); and **Enter**

**into Observer Mode** (Write off your weight, and journal or blog away your cravings).

- **D = Dream Big!** Then, **Do Sweet-Talk, Self-Talk, Affirmations, the Success Strut, My Simple 7 D's** (Delay, Distance, Distract, Decode, Decide, Diss, & Delight), and/or the **Sweeter, Full-Life Process** as well as **Tapping** (EFT) and **Metta Meditation** (*May I be safe, May I be happy, May I be healthy, May I live with ease*).

- **S = Seek Support** online and in person (from groups, loved ones, and professionals); **Sleep Enough; Savor the Flavors** and the **Sweetness of Doing Nothing; Shower Yourself with Love** and **Self-Compassion;** and **Say** *I'm sorry, Please forgive me, Thank you, I love you* (Ho'oponopono).

And always remember, this is *your* program. Claim it. Own it. Use it with pride, passion, and compassion.

I'm so excited for you. Let me heartily congratulate you on completing your six-week Beyond Sugar Shock program. Just imagine that I'm giving you a big celebratory hug and huge smile.  You did it! I knew you would!


## Before You Head into Your SWEETER Life, Have You Found Joy, Passion, and Spirit?

- Are you filling up at least several times a week on Sweet Relief Goodies such as Zumba, intenSati, Nia, or Masala Bhangra? Or have you found other activities that you like better?

- Are you giving yourself compassion every day?

- If you've slipped—or if you're tempted—are you repeating the Metta phrases and doing the other recommended tactics?

- Are you pursuing your passions so you can *Get Your Fill Now?* What are your new favorite passions?

- Have you set aside a special day to Savor the Sweetness of Doing Nothing? What are your plans? How do you Savor the Sweetness of Doing Nothing every day?

- Are you doing My Sweeter, Full-Life Process? How does it make you feel?

- Do you keep your Smart M.E.D.S. list in your wallet or phone so you can quickly get ideas to stay on track?

- Are you beginning to enjoy the bounty of a richer, sweeterlicious life?

I'm happy for you. This is the beginning of a joyous new life.

# SWEETEN YOUR LIFE NATURALLY & MOVE TOWARD A PLEASURABLE, PEACEFUL, SWEETERLICIOUS LIFE

### Affirmation: I have a sweeterlicious
### life full of passion, pleasure, and purpose.

Letting go of your addiction to refined sweets and culprit carbs and releasing your excess weight mark the beginning. You're now on your way to getting a more joyous, fulfilling, enriching life full of happiness, passion, pleasure, joy, and inner peace. What's more, you're now focused on creating a harmonious Mind-Body-Spirit balance.

*Beyond Sugar Shock* has given you a road map filled with practical and simple tools. Now it's up to you to create your own magnificent life and *Get a Life That Rocks*.

I invite you to continue to explore the lessons you've learned in this book and share them with your loved ones and friends. And if cravings strike or you need emotional or spiritual nourishment, just return to this book to get reacquainted with the cutting-edge techniques shared here so you can continue to access your inner peace and higher self.

You may even want to retake the Sugar Shock Quiz, or revisit it again in six months to see how much further you have moved Beyond Sugar Shock and how self-actualized you've become.

You're now ready for life's unexpected challenges. You can graciously accept and rise above them.

And remember: your frustrations, annoyances, or challenges can and will help you grow in ways you may have never imagined. As you continue to spurn those toxic carbs and grow spiritually, you'll find, as have Sugar Kickers worldwide, that you'll feel filled up in ways that once eluded you.

## What's Your Super Sweet Dream?

Now that you've released your sugar and carb addiction, you can focus on what *really* matters—your relationship with yourself, your loved ones, and the Universe, as well as with your enriching, rewarding passions. Instead of obsessing about sweets or carbs, you can set your sights on your *bold dreams and goals*—perhaps ones you've been ignoring for years.

Would you like to start or expand your family, take up painting and sell your work online, do stand-up comedy, launch an Internet business, do meaningful volunteer work, spend more time with your kids or husband, or write books and become a transformational speaker like me?

Whatever it is, go after it with all your energy, enthusiasm, and gusto.

Please stay in touch, too. Connect with us on Facebook, in my Beyond Sugar Shock Freedom Team on SparkPeople, or my Sugar Shock Blog.

Let us know how you're doing. Tell us about your passions and projects so we can support you, cheer you on, and spread the word to our many friends around the world about the awesome things you're creating.

In the meantime, enjoy your amazing, dazzling, sweeterlicious, new life.

# SHOP TO MOVE BEYOND SUGAR SHOCK

*"It's difficult to think anything but pleasant thoughts while eating a homegrown tomato."*

—AMERICAN WRITER AND HUMORIST LEWIS GRIZZARD (1946–1994)

It's time to go shopping for real, alive, nutrient-dense, seasonal quality foods. But before you go to the supermarket or farmers' market, take a close look at this Beyond Sugar Shock Shopping List.

Always keep healthy, local foods on hand. That way, no matter what, you'll always make smart, fiber-filled food choices.

By the way, although ideally you'll mostly select Mother Nature's fresh carb foods that grow on trees or out of the ground, or get grass-fed, free-range meats, you still can find some better prepared foods in boxes, cans, or jars. (Get a list of these superior packaged foods at my website.)

## VEGETARIAN PROTEIN

### Beans and Legumes
(Serving size = ½ cup.)

Adzuki
Black beans
Black-eyed peas
Broad beans
Butter beans
Garbanzo beans (also known as chickpeas)
Edamame beans* (also called soybeans)—preferably only twice a month
Fava beans
Great northern beans

Kidney beans
Lentils
Lima beans
Miso
Moth beans
Red beans
Refried beans
Soybeans* (also called edamame)
Split peas
Tempeh* (only twice a month)
Tofu, firm
White beans
Winged beans
Yellow beans

*Caution about soy:* Please note that soy is one of the top five food allergen/sensitivity foods, so it's not a good idea to consume a lot of this controversial fare. Most soy products are junk food—they're not traditional soy food (miso, tempeh, and the actual beans) that may have some slight positive effect on health. In fact, nutrition expert and exercise physiologist Jill Lane, C.N.C., who developed the Beyond Sugar Shock Meal Plan, doesn't recommend frequent consumption of soy in any form, because of the negative impact it can have on your thyroid. If you have a thyroid disease, you especially want to avoid consuming processed soy.

## NUTS AND SEEDS

*Caution:* About 1.3 percent of the general population may be allergic to peanuts, Brazil nuts, hazelnuts, walnuts, and almonds, which can cause anaphylactic shock. For nut butters, please choose organic, if possible.

**(Serving size = 10–12 nuts [maximum ¼ cup]. Serving size = 2 level tablespoons for nut butter.)**
Almond butter
Almonds
Brazil nuts
Cashew butter
Chia seeds

Coconut, natural (shredded and unsweetened)
Coconut milk, unsweetened**
Hazelnuts
Hickory nuts
Macadamia nut butter
Macadamia nuts
Peanut butter
Peanuts (considered nuts, but they're really legumes)
Pecans
Pistachios
Pumpkin and squash seeds
Sunflower seed kernels
Sesame seeds
Tahini (sesame seed spread)
Walnuts

**Please note that coconut milk comes from grinding up the coconut pulp and adding water. It's not *coconut water*, which has become increasingly popular. Coconut water has naturally occurring sugar in it, and 8 ounces is the equivalent of 1 piece of fruit.

### YOU'RE A HAPPY, SUCCESSFUL SUGAR KICKER WHEN . . .

You bring a BPA-free water bottle with you wherever you go. You'd rather take swigs of water instead of buying sodas, lemonade, or other sugary beverages.

## DAIRY PRODUCTS

*Caution about dairy:* About 75 percent of people are lactose intolerant. Some 30 million to 50 million Americans experience intestinal discomfort after consuming dairy products, with such symptoms as nausea, cramps, bloating, gas, diarrhea, and other painful gastrointestinal symptoms. If you have problems with cow's milk products, you may still be able to tolerate eggs or goat milk products. I recommend that you stick with organics for milk and yogurt.

**(Serving size = 1 ounce unless otherwise noted.)**
Blue cheese
Brie
Cheddar
Colby
Cottage cheese (½ cup)
Feta
Goat cheese, hard or soft
Gouda
Jarlsberg
Monterey Jack
Mozzarella, part-skim
Muenster
Parmesan, grated or hard
Provolone
Ricotta, part skim
Romano
Swiss

**Milk, Yogurt**
**(Serving size = 8 ounces unless otherwise noted.)**

Buttermilk, cultured
Cow's milk, organic
Goat's milk
Lactaid, 1% fat
Yogurt, low fat, plain (6 ounces)

## MEAT & PROTEIN

*Caution about meat and protein:* I recommend only free-range, grass-fed, organic meat, which means the animals weren't given antibiotics or hormones. I also recommend that you choose organic eggs, if possible.

### Eggs
Whole large (1 egg)

### Meat
**(Serving size = 4 ounces unless otherwise noted. Tip: 3–4 ounces is generally the size of a deck of cards.)**

Beef sausage (1 piece)
Beef, ground, extra lean
Beef, round, bottom
Buffalo
Flank steak
Lamb
Liver
Pot roast
Steak (rib eye, porterhouse, T-bone, sirloin, tenderloin)
Veal

### Poultry
**(Serving size = 4 ounces unless otherwise noted, preferably without skin.)**
Chicken breast
Chicken cutlet
Chicken, ground, white meat only
Cornish hen
Duck
Turkey breast
Turkey, ground (white or dark meat)
Turkey sausage (1 ounce)
Pheasant
Quail

## SEAFOOD

*Caution about seafood:* Ideally, you'll avoid freshwater fish, because lakes and rivers are often polluted. Choose fish from the Pacific Ocean or Alaskan waters. Smaller, nonpredatory fish such as flounder, sole, pollock, catfish, halibut, and clams are best. Eat sparingly of big fish such as swordfish, tuna, and shark, because these long-lived predatory fish tend to accumulate more mercury. Go to www.Beyond SugarShockFavorites.com to order from my favorite fish supplier, Vital Choice Seafood, which regularly tests fish to confirm that it's free of harmful contaminants such as mercury and PCBs.

**(Serving size = 4–6 ounces unless otherwise noted.)**
Abalone
Anchovy, fresh
Anchovy, canned in olive oil (5 anchovies)
Bass, striped
Bluefish
Catfish
Caviar, black and red
Clams
Cod
Crab, Alaska king or Dungeness
Crayfish
Flounder
Grouper
Haddock
Halibut
Herring
Lobster
Mackerel
Mussels, blue
Octopus
Orange Roughy
Oysters
Perch
Pike
Pompano

Salmon, fresh, Atlantic, Coho, wild Alaskan
Salmon, pink, canned
Sardines, canned in water (4 to 6 sardines)
Scallops, bay
Sea bass
Sea trout
Shrimp
Smelt
Snapper
Sole
Squid
Sturgeon
Swordfish
Trout, rainbow
Tuna, fresh, bluefin or yellowfin
Tuna, canned in spring water
Whitefish
Yellowtail

# FRUIT

*Smart Shopper Tip:* Pick from all colors of the rainbow and eat organic, if possible.

Apple (1 small/medium)
Apricots (3 medium)
Avocado (¼ medium)
Banana (½ medium)
Blackberries (1 cup)
Blueberries (¾ cup)
Boysenberries (1 cup)
Cantaloupe (1 cup)
Cherries (½ cup)
Crabapples (1 cup)
Cranberries (1 cup)
Figs (1 medium)
Gooseberries (1 cup)
Grapefruit (½ medium)

Grapes (1 cup)
Guava (1 medium)
Honeydew melon (1 cup)
Kiwi (1 medium)
Kumquats (1 medium)
Lychees (10 pieces)
Mango (½ cup)
Mulberries (1 cup)
Nectarine (1 small)
Orange (1 small)
Papaya (1 cup)
Passion fruit (1 medium)
Peach (1 medium)
Pear (1 medium)
Pineapple (¾ cup)
Plum (2 small)
Quince (1 medium)
Raspberries (1 cup)
Strawberries (1 cup or 6 berries)
Tangerine (1 medium)

## VEGETABLES

*Smart Shopper Tip:* If possible, eat organic produce.

**(Serving size = ½ cup cooked or 1 cup raw, unless otherwise noted. You want 4–6 servings a day.)**

Alfalfa sprouts
Artichoke (1 medium)
Arugula
Asparagus
Bamboo shoots
Bean Sprouts
Beets

Bok choy
Broccoli
Broccoli rabe
Brussels sprouts
Cabbage (all varieties)
Carrot
Cauliflower
Celeriac
Celery
Chicory
Collards
Cucumber
Eggplant
Endive
Fennel
Green beans
Jicama
Kale
Kohlrabi
Leeks
Lettuce, green or red leaf, radicchio, romaine, or mixed baby greens
Mushrooms
Mustard greens
Okra
Onions
Parsnips
Peppers, red, yellow, or green
Pumpkin
Radishes
Rhubarb
Rutabaga
Scallions
Snap peas
Spinach
Squash (all varieties)
Swiss chard
Tomato (1 medium)

Turnip
Turnip greens
Water chestnuts
Watercress
Yam/Sweet potatoes
Zucchini

## WHOLE GRAINS

*Caution about grains:* Before eating gluten-containing grains such as wheat, rye, spelt, and barley, you may want to find out if you have a gluten sensitivity or celiac disease, which means you're intolerant to these foods, as well as beer and ales. See information about celiac disease and gluten intolerance, cited previously. Gluten-free grains are: buckwheat, millet, oats and oat groats (if designated gluten-free), quinoa, brown rice or wild rice, sorghum, teff, and products from corn or beans. If you don't have gluten issues, these are some whole grains from which you can choose:

**(Serving size = ½ cup cooked, unless otherwise noted. Read labels carefully to make sure all items are sugar-free.)**

Barley
Bran
Bread, 100% whole-grain (1 slice)
Buckwheat
Bulgur
Cracked wheat
Crackers, whole-grain (5 crackers)
Durum wheat
Hard red winter wheat
Kamut
Kasha
Millet (¼ cup)
Muesli (¼ cup)
Oats and oat groats
Quinoa (½ cup)

Rice, brown (⅓ cup)
Rice, wild (⅓ cup)
Rye berries
Sorghum
Spelt
Teff
Wheat germ (3 tablespoons)
Wheat berries
Whole-wheat couscous
Whole-wheat pasta
Whole-wheat pita (6 inches or ½ pita)

# FATS

*Fat Pointers:* Superior fats are rich in monounsaturated fat, so eat those more often. If possible, always use organic, virgin oils. The best to cook with are olive oil, coconut oil, and macadamia nut oil. Coconut oil has been praised for being antimicrobial, a fat-loss tool, and a good energy source.

**(Serving size = 1 tablespoon unless otherwise noted.)**

Chia seeds
Coconut oil (best oil to use at high heat)
Flax seed oil (best to refrigerate/don't cook with it)
Flax seed meal (2 tablespoons per day is ideal)
Macadamia nut oil
Olive oil (good for dressings but if you cook with it, do so at a low to medium heat)
Olives (about 6 medium-sized)
Sesame oil (nice for salad dressings and stir-fry foods)

Other healthy fat choices include the nuts and nut butters mentioned above. For example, you could try 1 tablespoon of slivered almonds or 1 to 2 tablespoons of nut butter.

## HERBS AND SPICES

When you're cooking, spices are a great way to liven up your dishes—and get some benefits at the same time.

Basil
Bay leaf
Cayenne
Caraway
Chervil
Chive
Cinnamon*
Cloves*
Coriander*
Crushed pepper
Ground red pepper
Cumin
Curry
Dill
Fennel
Garlic
Ginger**
Marjoram
Mint
Mustard (dry)*
Nutmeg*
Oregano
Parsley
Paprika
Rosemary
Sage
Savory
Tarragon
Thyme
Turmeric**

*Cinnamon, cloves, and nutmeg increase insulin's ability to metabolize sugar and remove it from the blood, according to nutritionist Ann Louise Gittleman, Ph.D. In addition, coriander, dry mustard, and ginger lessen your risk of excess insulin by speeding up your metabolism or lowering glucose levels.

**Integrative Physician Andrew Weil, M.D. recommends both turmeric and ginger for anti-inflammatory support.

## SEA VEGETABLES (SEAWEED) & SEASONINGS

Arame
Dulse
Hijiki
Kelp
Laver
Nori
Wakame
Triple Blend Flakes (from Maine Coast)
Eden Organic Seaweed Gomasio

### Taste Treats from the Sea

If you're not a fan of seaweed, you're in for a real treat. These tasty sea veggies can add zest and flavor to salads, main courses, and more. You can use sea salt, especially low-sodium blends from Maine Coast, instead of regular salt. They're also high in minerals such as iodine.

## SUPERFOODS

Sprinkle a little, if you like, into morning or afternoon power smoothies. (You may wish to consume maca separately, though.)

Cacao beans or powder (real chocolate without sugar)
Chia Seeds
Maca
Goji Berries
Wild bee pollen
Marine phytoplankton

## CONDIMENTS, GARNISHES, AND SAUCES

*Caution about condiments:* Make sure none of these items contains added or hidden sugars.

Apple Cider Vinegar*
Capers
Dill pickles
Lemon juice*
Lime juice*
Marinara Sauce
Mustard
Olives
Roasted pepper
Salsa

*Using apple cider vinegar, or lemon or lime juice with meals helps you digest carbohydrates more slowly, which keeps your glucose levels stable and can lower your blood sugar by as much as 30 percent, according to Dr. Gittleman.

## BEVERAGES

**Water (filtered or spring)**
To make your water more enticing, see my SWEET Success Strategy on page 140.

**Herbal Teas** (Some of my favorites are listed below in alphabetical order by brand.)
- **Bigelow:** Mint Medley, Cozy Chamomile, etc.
- **Celestial Seasonings:** Tension Tamer, Mandarin Orange Spice, Almond Sunset, Ginkgo Sharp, etc.
- **Mighty Leaf:** Sanctuary, Renewal, Calming Moon, Chrysanthemum, Organic Berry Wellness, etc.
- **Tazo:** Sweet Cinnamon Spice, Wild Sweet Orange, Refresh, etc.
- **Traditional Medicinals:** Organic Cold Care P.M., Think-O2, Easy Now, Throat Coat, etc.
- **Yogi Tea:** Bedtime, Ginger, Calming, Ginkgo Clarity, Kava Stress Relief, Ginseng, Chamomile, Royal Vitality, Computer De-Stress Tea, Stomach Ease, Echinacea Immune Support, etc.

# MEAL PLAN & RECIPES TO MOVE YOU BEYOND SUGAR SHOCK

*"To eat is a necessity, but to eat intelligently is an art."*
— FRENCH AUTHOR FRANCOIS DE LA ROCHEFOUCAULD (1613–1680)

To get you started on your sweeterlicious journey, here are some simple, tasty meal plans and sugar-free recipes for one week.

You can find more meal plans and recipes by going to my website www .BeyondSugarShock.com.

Unless specified, recipes are from Jill Lane, C.N.C.

If you follow a special diet that's free of meat, gluten, or dairy, you can easily adapt recipes to work for your special diet. Please note that I recommend you go meatless on the first day of every week. The worldwide grassroots Meatless Monday movement (www.MeatlessMonday.com) is a nonprofit initiative of the Monday Campaigns, in association with the Johns Hopkins Bloomberg School of Public Health. The program urges you to reduce your meat consumption by 15 percent to improve your health (helping to reduce your risk of such chronic, preventable conditions as cancer, cardiovascular disease, and type 2 diabetes), save precious resources, and reduce your carbon footprint.

Recipes for items marked with an asterisk (*) can be found on pages 212–229.

For any foods on your meal plan, if you eat more than the recommended portion size and/or crave them when you're under stress or facing other emotional challenges, that could be a sign this is a trigger food for you. If that's the case, it may easier for you to not keep those particular foods in the house. For more information about trigger foods, read the article "Trigger Foods that Cause Binges" on my Sugar Shock Blog at www.SugarShockBlog.com.

## MEAL PLAN SAMPLE WEEK

### DAY 1

| | |
|---|---|
| **Breakfast** | Super Oatmeal* |
| | 2 hard-boiled, free-range eggs (3 for men or those who weigh more than 200 pounds) |
| **Lunch** | Greek Spinach Salad* |
| **Snack** | 2 Wasa Hearty Rye Crispbread crackers or 8–10 gluten-free Mary's Gone Crackers crackers with 3 tablespoons sugar-free salsa (optional) |
| **Dinner** | Stuffed Bell Peppers* |
| | 1 cup raw spinach side salad, with Olive Oil Dressing* |
| **Optional Evening Snack** | 1 small apple with 1–2 tablespoons almond or cashew butter |

### DAY 2

| | |
|---|---|
| **Breakfast** | Egg and Veggie Scramble* |
| | 1 slice no-sugar-added, whole-grain bread (if going gluten-free, substitute with another cup fruit) |
| | 1 cup sliced strawberries |
| **Lunch** | Avocado Chicken Salad* |
| **Snack** | 2 organic celery stalks |
| | 3 tablespoons hummus |
| **Dinner** | Connie's Mustard-Dill Salmon* |
| | 1½ cups Jill's Herby Tomato Salad* |
| | 6 stalks roasted asparagus |
| | ½ cup wild rice or 1 skewer of Connie's Frozen Fruit Kabobs* (optional) |
| **Optional Evening Snack** | ¼ cup raw shelled sunflower seeds |
| | ½ pear |

## MEAL PLAN SAMPLE WEEK

### DAY 3

| | |
|---|---|
| Breakfast | 4 small organic turkey or chicken breakfast sausages |
| | 1 slice sugar-free, whole-grain or gluten-free bread |
| | 1–2 tablespoons almond or cashew butter |
| Lunch | Tuna Broccoli Slaw* |
| Snack | 2 tablespoons hummus |
| | ½ cucumber, sliced |
| Dinner | Turkey or Bison Burger* and Mexican Green Salad* |
| Optional Evening Snack | 3 ounces nitrate-free deli meat or 1 hardboiled egg wrapped in a lettuce leaf |

### DAY 4

| | |
|---|---|
| Breakfast | 2 omega-3 enriched, free-range hardboiled eggs (3 for men) |
| | ½ grapefruit (or other fruit of your choice) |
| Lunch | Roasted Turkey Wrap* |
| | 2 organic celery stalks |
| | 2 tablespoons guacamole |
| Snack | Connie's Crispy Kale Chips* |
| Dinner | Veggie and Chicken Kabobs* |
| | ⅓ cup Walnut Rosemary Quinoa Pilaf* (optional) |
| Optional Evening Snack | ¾ cup unsalted edamame (served hot or cold) |

### DAY 5

| | |
|---|---|
| Breakfast | Super Oatmeal* |
| | 4 organic turkey or chicken breakfast sausage links |
| Lunch | Chef's Salad* |
| Snack | 1 orange |
| | 12–15 raw nuts of your choice |
| Dinner | Sea Scallops* and Sautéed Spinach with Garlic* |
| | ⅓ cup Walnut Rosemary Quinoa Pilaf* (optional) |
| Optional Evening Snack | Connie's Crispy Kale Chips* |

## MEAL PLAN SAMPLE WEEK

### DAY 6

| | |
|---|---|
| **Breakfast** | 3 strips organic turkey bacon |
| | 1 unsweetened brown rice cake |
| | 1 tablespoon almond or cashew butter |
| **Lunch** | Egg Salad* |
| **Snack** | 1 cup berries |
| | 2 tablespoons pumpkin seeds |
| **Dinner** | Steak* and Jill's Roasted Veggies* |
| | 2 cups raw spinach, topped with slivered almonds, and mixed with 1½ tablespoons Olive Oil Dressing* |
| **Optional Evening Snack** | 1 cup berries |
| | 12 raw nuts or 3 tablespoons sugar-free coconut milk yogurt |

### DAY 7

| | |
|---|---|
| **Breakfast** | Egg and Veggie Scramble* |
| | 1 slice Mestemacher Fitness Bread or 1 slice French Meadow Health-seed Spelt Bread. (If avoiding gluten, add another cup of berries or 1 slice gluten-free bread) |
| | 1 cup sliced strawberries |
| **Lunch** | 1 cup organic cottage cheese (replace with 1 can drained water-packed tuna if you're avoiding dairy) served on mixed green salad: 1½ cups combined chopped tomato, cucumber, red and yellow peppers; ¼ sliced avocado; ½ cup cooked black beans; 1 tablespoon olive oil; and black pepper to taste |
| **Snack** | 1 unsweetened brown rice cake |
| | 1–2 tablespoons almond or cashew butter |
| **Dinner** | Dijon Shrimp* |
| | ½ medium sweet potato, roasted or baked (optional) |
| | 3 cups mixed green salad with Olive Oil Dressing* |
| **Optional Evening Snack** | ¼ medium avocado |
| | 3 tablespoons sugar-free salsa |

## RECIPES (Listed in Alphabetical Order)

Avocado Chicken Salad

Balsamic Dressings

Bison Burger (See Turkey Burger)

Chef's Salad

Connie's Crispy Kale Chips

Connie's Frozen Fruit Kabobs

Connie's Mustard-Dill Salmon

Connie's Super-Simple Chia-Flax-Lemon Salad Dressing

Dijon Shrimp

Egg and Veggie Scramble

Egg Salad

Greek Spinach Salad

Jill's Herby Tomato Salad

Jill's Roasted Veggies

Mexican Green Salad

Olive Oil Dressings

Roasted Turkey Wrap

Sautéed Spinach with Garlic

Sea Scallops

Steak

Stuffed Bell Peppers (Meatless Monday Option)

Super Oatmeal

Tuna Broccoli Slaw

Turkey or Bison Burger

Veggie and Chicken Kabobs

Walnut Rosemary Quinoa Pilaf (Meatless Monday Option)

## AVOCADO CHICKEN SALAD

Preparation time: 5–10 minutes

    2 cups mixed greens
    ½ tomato, sliced
    ½ cucumber
    ½ red and yellow peppers, seeded and ribs removed
    ¼ medium avocado, sliced or diced
    ½ cup chickpeas
    4 ounces chicken breast, skinless and boneless, cooked and sliced
    2 tablespoons Olive Oil Dressing of your choice (page 222)

Mix all the vegetables and top with chicken and salad dressing.

*1 serving*

## BALSAMIC DRESSINGS

Preparation time: about 10 minutes

> 1 tablespoon Dijon mustard
> ¼ cup balsamic vinegar
> ½ cup extra-virgin, cold-pressed olive oil*

Whisk together mustard and vinegar. While mixing, slowly add the oil. Serve immediately or chill for later use. Add additional mustard or vinegar to suit your individual taste.

* If you want to improve the fatty acid ratio of this dressing, use 6 tablespoons of olive oil plus 2 tablespoons of flax oil.

*6 servings*

**Variations:** Any of the following ingredients may be added while blending the Dijon and vinegar:

Fresh herbs such as basil, cilantro, rosemary, parsley, oregano, or thyme

Fresh minced garlic

Chopped shallots or onions

Sun-dried tomatoes

Fresh cracked pepper

Feta or goat cheese

## CHEF'S SALAD

Preparation time: 5 minutes

- 2 cups mixed greens
- 4 ounces (6 for men) shredded all-natural, low-sodium turkey or chicken deli slices (or you can crumble a turkey burger)
- 2 cups chopped veggies of choice (recommendations include: tomato, bell peppers, Peperoncini peppers, olives, cucumber, zucchini, broccoli, and mushrooms)
- 2 tablespoons dressing of choice (pages 213, 218, or 222)

Mix ingredients together in a medium bowl. Add dressing.

*1 serving*

## CONNIE'S CRISPY KALE CHIPS

Cooking time: 5–10 minutes

- 1 head kale, washed, with the bottoms cut off and the leaves pulled into large pieces
- 1 tablespoon coconut oil
- Dash of Maine Coast Kelp Granules, Dulse Flakes, and/or Eden Organic's Gomasio
- 2–3 pieces of SeaSnax or other nori seaweed

Dip kale into coconut oil in a large frying pan, making sure the leaves are lightly oiled.

Sprinkle on Maine Coast Kelp Granules, Dulse Flakes and/or some Eden Organic's Gomasio. Add a few pieces of SeaSnax or other nori seaweed.

Heat the frying pan with the kale at the lowest possible heat. Turn kale over several times. Cook until crisp.

**Note:** You can also use additional spices like turmeric, cayenne, dill weed, or cumin if you'd like more kick.

*3 servings*

## CONNIE'S FROZEN FRUIT KABOBS

Preparation time: 20 minutes
Freezing time: about 2 hours

> 4 bamboo skewers
> 4–5 of the following fruits; choose fruits that are in season:
> > 12 large strawberries, preferably organic, cored and halved
> > 1 ripe pear (Anjou, Bartlett, Red Bartlett, or Asian), peeled and cut into bite-sized pieces
> > 8 purple or green grapes
> > 20 blueberries
> > 2 plums, peeled and cut into bite-sized pieces
> > 2 peaches, peeled and cut into bite-sized pieces
> > 12 raspberries or blackberries
> > 8 cherries, halved
> > ¼ banana*
> Cinnamon, to taste
> Cacao nibs (unsweetened)
> 4 teaspoons finely chopped walnuts (optional)
> 4 teaspoons unsweetened shredded coconut (optional)

Clean all the fruit, and split into four batches, with some of each fruit in every batch. Slide the fruit onto the four skewers, alternating fruits.

Place the skewers onto a large metal pan, and put them in freezer for about 2 hours. Freeze longer if you wish.

When fruit has reached desired consistency sprinkle with cinnamon and cacao. Add walnuts and shredded coconut, if desired. Eat immediately or freeze for later (simply remove from freezer 5–15 minutes before you want to eat them).

**Note:** This dessert is great to eat if you're craving sorbet, ice cream, or a Popsicle. Tell us on my Facebook fan page (www.Facebook.com/SmartHabitsFans) how your Frozen Fruit Kabobs saved you from dangerous sweets.

*Bananas take longer to freeze than the other fruits.

*4 servings*

## CONNIE'S MUSTARD-DILL SALMON

Cooking time: about 20 minutes

> 2 teaspoons extra-virgin olive oil
> Two 4-ounce salmon fillets
> Juice from 2 lemons
> 1½ tablespoons stone-ground mustard (or to taste)
> 2 to 4 teaspoons capers
> 2 tablespoons chopped dill
> Dash of cilantro (optional)

Preheat oven to 400 degrees, and use oil to lightly oil a baking sheet.

Place salmon on the baking sheet.

Squeeze lemon on salmon. Slather with mustard, top with capers, and sprinkle liberally with dill. Add cilantro, if desired.

Grill or broil salmon for about 20 minutes in oven, or until just opaque in the center.

*2 servings*

## CONNIE'S SUPER-SIMPLE CHIA-FLAX-LEMON SALAD DRESSING

Preparation time: 3 minutes

Juice of 2–3 lemons, to taste
¼ cup filtered water
½ cup extra-virgin, cold-pressed olive oil or flax oil
Sesame seeds, to taste
Chia seeds, to taste
Ground flax seeds, to taste
Sea salt or seaweed such as dulse and nori, to taste

Combine all ingredients in a blender and mix until fully combined. Serve at once or refrigerate for later use. Add additional lemon juice and water to make the dressing less thick.

*5 servings*


## DIJON SHRIMP

Cooking time: about 10 minutes

8 ounces cleaned large shrimp
2 tablespoons coconut oil or extra-virgin olive oil
1 clove garlic, minced
1 cup no-sugar-added marinara sauce
1 tablespoon Dijon mustard

Sauté or grill shrimp in 1½ tablespoons oil until cooked through. Set aside.

Cook garlic in 1/2 tablespoon oil in sauté pan over medium heat, add marinara sauce and mustard. Add shrimp and stir for 2–3 minutes.

*2 servings*

## EGG AND VEGGIE SCRAMBLE

Cooking time: 10–12 minutes

    2 tablespoons extra-virgin olive oil
    1 cup fresh vegetables, washed, chopped (choose a mix of your own favorites,
      such as: broccoli, spinach, mushroom, tomato, onion, and bell pepper)
    2 organic eggs (3 eggs for men)
    Sea salt and pepper, to taste

Heat oil in a small frying pan over a medium heat. Add vegetables and stir occasionally.

Cook about 5–6 minutes, or until they reach desired consistency.

Meanwhile, lightly whip eggs with a fork in a bowl.

Pour eggs over vegetables in pan. Stir mixture lightly with a fork, until the eggs are thoroughly cooked, about 5 minutes. Add salt and pepper to taste.

*1 serving*

## EGG SALAD

Cooking time: about 12 minutes

    6 eggs
    One 6-inch stalk organic celery, chopped
    ¼ cup chopped green onion (optional)
    2 tablespoons plain yogurt (if avoiding dairy, use canola mayonnaise)
    2 tablespoons olive oil
    1 teaspoon black pepper
    1 teaspoon paprika
    ½ teaspoon sea salt

Hard-boil the eggs for 12 minutes. Cool and dice, then mix with the remaining ingredients.

*2 servings*

## GREEK SPINACH SALAD

Preparation time: 5 minutes

    2 cups fresh spinach, rinsed and chopped
    1 cup chickpeas, canned or cooked
    ½ cucumber, sliced
    ½ cup diced tomato
    4–6 chopped olives
    1½ tablespoons Olive Oil Dressing (page 222)

Mix spinach with the other ingredients in medium bowl. Top with salad dressing.

*1 serving*


## JILL'S HERBY TOMATO SALAD

Preparation time: 5 minutes

    1 package cherry or plum tomatoes, or 4 Roma tomatoes, diced
    ½ cucumber, peeled and diced
    ¼ red onion, diced
    2–3 tablespoons extra-virgin olive oil
    1 tablespoon each of fresh chopped cilantro, basil, and parsley
    1 tablespoon lemon zest
    2–3 tablespoons apple-cider vinegar
    Sea salt and pepper, to taste

Toss tomatoes, cucumbers, and onion in bowl with olive oil, fresh chopped herbs, and lemon zest.

Toss with apple-cider vinegar. Add salt and pepper to taste.

*2–3 servings*

## JILL'S ROASTED VEGGIES

Cooking time: about 15–20 minutes

> 4 cups (chopped or sliced into bite-sized pieces) vegetables
> from the following list:
>> Asparagus
>> Bell peppers (green, red, or yellow)
>> Broccoli
>> Cauliflower
>> Green beans
>> Mushrooms
>> Squash (green or yellow)
>> Yams, sweet potatoes, or butternut squash (for root veggies,
>> roast 10 minutes
>> prior to adding the rest)
>> Zucchini
> 2–3 garlic cloves, minced
> 2 tablespoons extra-virgin olive oil
> Sea salt, to taste
> Paprika, to taste
> Garlic powder, to taste
> Turmeric, to taste
> Cracked black pepper, to taste

Preheat oven to 400 degrees.

In a large bowl, toss veggies and garlic with the oil.

Spread on a large sheet pan and roast at 400 degrees on the top rack for 15–20 minutes (or to desired tenderness).

Set aside at room temperature for 2–5 minutes, then season to taste with any combination of the spices listed above.

*2 servings*

## MEXICAN GREEN SALAD

Preparation time: 5 minutes

> 3 cups mixed greens
> 2 tablespoons each of pumpkin seeds, chopped jicama, and fresh cilantro
> 1/2 cup cooked black beans (optional)
> 2 tablespoons no-sugar-added salsa (get my recipe at www
>     .BeyondSugarShock.com)
> 1 tablespoon extra-virgin olive oil

Toss ingredients together in a medium bowl.

*1 serving*

## OLIVE OIL DRESSING

Preparation time: 5 minutes

> ½ cup extra-virgin, cold-pressed olive oil
> 1 tablespoon Dijon mustard, or to taste

Whisk together oil and mustard until well combined. Serve at once or refrigerate for later use.

\* If you want to improve the fatty acid ratio of this dressing, use 6 tablespoons of olive oil plus 2 tablespoons of flax oil.

*4 servings*

**Variations:** To enhance and/or change the flavor, you may add any of the following ingredients to the oil-and-mustard mixture while blending:

Fresh herbs such as basil, cilantro, rosemary, parsley, oregano, or thyme

Fresh minced garlic

Chopped shallots or green onions

Sun-dried tomatoes

Fresh cracked pepper

## ROASTED TURKEY WRAP

Preparation time: 5 minutes

- 4 ounces (5–6 ounces for men) roasted turkey, sliced
- 4–6 whole red leaf or butter lettuce leaves, chopped
- 1 tomato, sliced
- 2 teaspoons no-sugar-added mustard
- 1 whole-wheat tortilla (If avoiding gluten, use lettuce leaves for wraps instead of the tortilla)

Mix the first four ingredients in bowl. Spoon the mix into the tortilla.

*1 serving*

## SAUTÉED SPINACH WITH GARLIC

Cooking time: about 6 minutes

- 1½ tablespoons extra-virgin olive oil
- 1 garlic clove, minced
- ½ teaspoon cracked red pepper (optional)
- 2 cups (big handfuls) spinach, rinsed and patted dry

Heat oil in frying pan over medium-low heat.

Add garlic and red pepper, and cook until garlic is lightly browned.

Add spinach and sauté for about 3–4 minutes.

*1 serving*

## SEA SCALLOPS

Preparation time: 30 minutes
Cooking time: about 4 minutes

> Juice from 1 lemon and 1 lime
> 1 teaspoons dried basil or 2 teaspoons finely chopped fresh basil
> 1 teaspoons dried parsley or 2 teaspoons finely chopped fresh parsley
> 4–5 ounces sea scallops
> 2 teaspoons olive oil

In a zippered plastic bag, mix citrus juice with herbs.

Add scallops and marinate for 30 minutes.

Heat oil in a frying pan over medium-high heat. Add scallops and cook until brown, about 2 minutes per side.

*1 serving*

## STEAK

Cooking time: 10–16 minutes

> 4 ounces lean steak (such as filet, flank, or NY strip)
> 1 tablespoon extra-virgin olive oil
> ½ teaspoon black pepper
> ½ teaspoon dried rosemary
> ¼ teaspoon sea salt

Rub or brush steak with mixture of oil, pepper, rosemary, and sea salt.

Broil or grill steak for 5–8 minutes on each side, for medium. For well-done, cook longer.

*1 serving*

## STUFFED BELL PEPPERS
## (MEATLESS MONDAY OPTION)

Reprinted, courtesy of Alexandra Jamieson (www.deliciousvitality.com)

Cooking time: 25 minutes

- 1 teaspoon extra-virgin olive oil
- 2 bell peppers, red or green, sliced in half, leaving stem intact so the halves hold their shape during cooking, seeds and ribs removed
- One 14.5-ounce can black beans, rinsed and drained
- ½ cup shredded carrot
- 1 tablespoon fresh lime juice
- 1 garlic clove, minced
- 1 tablespoon chopped fresh cilantro
- 1 tablespoon chopped fresh flat-leaf parsley
- 1 cup chopped tomatoes
- ½ cup corn kernels
- ¼ cup sliced green onions
- ¼ teaspoon cayenne
- ½ teaspoon ground cumin
- Sea salt and pepper, to taste

Preheat oven to 350 degrees. Use oil to lightly oil a small baking dish.

Set aside pepper halves. Combine remaining ingredients in a mixing bowl and toss well.

Fill peppers with the mixture, place in baking dish, and fill baking dish with ¼ inch water.

Cover baking dish with foil and bake for 15 minutes.

Remove foil and bake for another 10 minutes.

*2 servings*

## SUPER OATMEAL

Preparation time: 3 minutes

    ¾ cup cooked steel-cut oatmeal
    1 tablespoon ground golden flax seeds or 8 chopped walnuts
    1 teaspoon cinnamon or pumpkin pie spice
    3 tablespoons organic 2% milk, *or* unsweetened rice or almond milk (optional)

Top oatmeal with flax seeds or walnuts, and cinnamon or pumpkin pie spice.

If desired, add milk for moisture. If you're avoiding dairy, use rice or almond milk.

*1 serving*

## TUNA BROCCOLI SLAW

Preparation time: 3 minutes

    One 6-ounce can water-packed tuna
    2 cups broccoli slaw
    ⅓ cup chopped tomato
    ⅓ cup cooked kidney beans
    2 tablespoons Olive Oil Dressing

Toss ingredients together in a medium bowl.

If you choose, you may use sesame oil in place of olive oil in dressing recipe. Pour over salad.

*1 serving*

## TURKEY OR BISON BURGER

Cooking time: 10–15 minutes

> 1 pound ground turkey or bison
> ½ cup chopped yellow or green onion
> 2 tablespoons Dijon mustard
> 1–2 teaspoons black pepper (optional)
> 2 teaspoons garlic powder (optional)
> 1 teaspoon sea salt (optional)
> 2 teaspoons olive oil to coat pan
> Trimmings: sliced, sugar-free pickles, tomatoes, and sprouts or lettuce

Place meat in a bowl. Add onion, mustard, and spices, and combine.

Shape mixture into 4 patties.

Grill or pan-cook turkey burgers, for about 7 minutes on one side, then flip and cook for about 5 minutes for medium or more for well-done. For bison burgers, cook about 5 minutes on each side, again according to preference.

Serve with trimmings.

3–4 servings

## VEGGIE AND CHICKEN KABOBS

Cooking time: about 20–30 minutes

> 2–3 wood or bamboo skewers, presoaked in water
> One 4- to 5-ounce boneless, skinless chicken breast, cut into 1½-inch cubes
> 1 green or red bell pepper, seeds and ribs removed, sliced into chunks
> 1 yellow squash, sliced into ¼- to ½-inch-thick rounds
> 1 zucchini, sliced into ¼- to ½-inch-thick rounds
> 10 cherry tomatoes
> 2 teaspoons extra-virgin olive oil
> Sea salt and pepper, to taste

Fill 2–3 skewers by alternating chicken and veggies.

Drizzle skewers with olive oil and sprinkle with salt and pepper.

Place on hot grill. Cook until juices run clear in chicken, and veggies are tender—approximately 20 minutes.

*1 serving*

## WALNUT ROSEMARY QUINOA PILAF
## (MEATLESS MONDAY OPTION)

Reprinted, courtesy of http://www.savvyvegetarian.com

Cooking time: 30 minutes

- 1 tablespoon extra-virgin olive oil
- 1 small onion, diced (optional)
- 2 cloves garlic, minced
- 1 medium carrot, peeled and diced
- 1 stalk celery, diced
- 1 cup quinoa, rinsed
- ½ teaspoon dried rosemary or 1 teaspoon fresh chopped rosemary
- 1 bay leaf
- 1 unsalted vegetable bouillon cube *or* 1 teaspoon sugar-free bouillon powder
- ½ teaspoon sea salt (optional)
- Fresh ground pepper, to taste (optional)
- ½ cup chopped unsalted walnuts, soaked in water for 6 hours or longer
- ¼ cup parsley (optional)
- ½ cup of fresh or frozen peas or ½ cup of cooked chick peas (optional)

Heat oil in a sauté pan and add onion, garlic, carrot, and celery. Sauté over medium heat, while stirring constantly for 3 minutes. Add quinoa, rosemary, bay leaf, bouillon, salt, and pepper, and sauté an additional 2 minutes.

Add 1½ cups boiling water and bring mixture back to a boil. Then cover, reduce heat, and simmer for 15 minutes.

When the quinoa is cooked, turn off the heat and mix in the walnuts, plus parsley and peas or chickpeas.

Let sit covered for an additional 10 minutes before serving.

*4 servings*

## SNACK LIST

These are optional. If you have hypoglycemia or low blood sugar, two snacks per day may be just what you need. (That's the case with me.) Try not to go longer than four hours without eating, and don't eat within two to three hours before bedtime.

- ¼ cup homemade raw nut trail mix: Take 1 tablespoon no-sugar-added dried fruit and 2 tablespoons raw nut of choice, mix together, and enjoy. (*NOTE:* Some of my clients find it challenging to eat dried fruit, because it triggers sugar cravings. If so, choose another snack.)

- 8–10 ounces low-sodium or homemade vegetable juice and 10 raw nuts

- 2 deviled eggs or 1–2 hard-boiled eggs (with yolks), with tomato slices, or other assorted veggies

- 1 cup sliced veggies (such as cucumbers, celery, broccoli, jicama, or zucchini) with ½ cup hummus as dip

- 2 tablespoons almond butter *or* 1 tablespoon egg salad or hummus split between four 3-inch celery sticks

- ½ cucumber with 2 tablespoons peanut butter

- 10–15 raw nuts (walnuts, almonds, or pistachios) with 1 cup or 1 piece fruit of your choice

- 1–2 cups of Connie's Crispy Kale Chips, with 1 hard-boiled egg

- 3 ounces low-sodium deli turkey or chicken, with 4 baby carrots

- ¾ cup edamame

- 2 tablespoons almond butter split between wedges of 1 small apple

- Yogurt parfait (plain, unsweetened, organic yogurt—use goat's or coconut yogurt, if desired), 2 tablespoons slivered almonds *or* flax seed meal, and ½ cup berries

- 1 mozzarella string cheese stick, with 1 apple, orange, pear, or ¾ cup fresh berries. (Choose a different snack if you're not having dairy.)

- 2–3 ounces organic, low-sodium, no-sugar-added chicken or turkey deli meat slices, each spread with 2 teaspoons cream cheese, goat cheese, or hummus, and topped with 1 small sugar-free dill pickle spear, rolled up

# SUPPLEMENTS TO CURB YOUR CRAVINGS & EASE YOU INTO THE LAND OF SUGAR-FREE

People often ask me what supplements can help quell their carb cravings. Of course you'll want to see a medical professional first, but ideally you'll first take a high-quality, professional-grade multivitamin/mineral with no iron (unless recommended by your doctor).

Next, you can calm your cravings with chromium; a high-quality, clean, professional-grade fish oil (from anchovy, sardine, mackerel, krill, or cod); and L-glutamine powder. You also can get more cravings support from 5HTP (but do *not* take if you're on an SSRI antidepressant or MAOI drug), vanadium, and B Complex (which you never want to take at dinner, because it can energize you). And if you have insulin resistance, alpha-lipoic acid, biotin, Acetyl-L-Carnitine, and GLA can help you, according to Jill Lane, C.N.C.

Overwhelmed by all these options? To make it easy for you and to save you money, we're offering a Beyond Sugar Shock Freedom Success Kit (containing several supplements), the Super-Duper Sugar Freedom Success Kit, a Vegetarian Sugar Freedom Success Kit, Beyond Sugar Shock Fat-Release Kit, and others. Get info at my website, www.BeyondSugarShock.com.

**Disclosure:** These supplement suggestions and statements have not been evaluated by the Food and Drug Administration (FDA). These are not intended to diagnose, treat, cure, or prevent any disease.

**YOU'RE A HAPPY, SUCCESSFUL SUGAR KICKER WHEN . . .**
You take supplements to help calm your cravings and balance your blood sugar levels.

# REMARKABLE RESOURCES TO RELAX, REFRESH & HEAL YOU

*"Physician, heal thyself."*
— LUKE 4:23

To help you reach a sweeterlicious place of Mind-Body-Spirit wholeness, I encourage you to rely on some of my favorite resources. Learn more about all of these products, services, and programs at my website www.BeyondSugarShock.com. Just click on the Resources tab to get more information and links.

## BOOKS

I recommend so many books, CDs, and DVDs that I've set up a special bookstore page on my website. Some of my favorites (as I write this) include:

- *The 150 Healthiest Foods on Earth* by Jonny Bowden, Ph.D.

- *The Art of Extreme Self-Care* by Cheryl Richardson

- *Beat Sugar Addiction Now!: The Cutting-Edge Program That Cures Your Type of Sugar Addiction and Puts You on the Road to Feeling Great—and Losing Weight!* by Jacob Teitelbaum, M.D.

- *A Course in Weight Loss* by Marianne Williamson

- *The End of Overeating* by David Kessler, M.D.

- *Get the Sugar Out* and *Zapped* by Ann Louise Gittleman, Ph.D.

- *The Map* by Colette Baron-Reid

- *Saved by an Angel* by Doreen Virtue

- *Self Compassion: Stop Beating Yourself Up and Leave Insecurity Behind* by Kristin Neff, Ph.D.

- *The Self-Compassion Diet* by Jean Fain
- *Suicide by Sugar* by Nancy Appleton, Ph.D.
- *Wherever You Go, There You Are* by Jon Kabat-Zinn, Ph.D.
- *You Can Create an Exceptional Life* by Louise Hay and Cheryl Richardson

I also recommend the riveting films *The Tapping Solution, What the Bleep Do We Know, Under Our Skin, You Can Heal Your Life, King Corn, Bag It, The Secret,* and *Full Signal.* Get more suggestions and links in the Book Store section of my websites.

## EARTHING OR GROUNDING

All of us, by using cell phones, computers, PDAs, wireless routers, fluorescent lights, and other technological devices, are being exposed to massive amounts of potentially harmful electromagnetic fields (EMFs)—as much as 100 million times more electromagnetic radiation than our grandparents faced. Because of this invisible electropollution, we're potentially vulnerable to a host of health problems. Researchers have even discovered that EMFs can result in type 3 diabetes, as researchers call it, in people extra sensitive to electrical devices that emit "dirty" electricity. The good news is that scientists have developed *earthing* or *grounding*, which helps you tap into the earth's natural healing energies through conductive body bands, bed-sheets, and floor mats. Studies show that earthing may reduce inflammation, improve your sleep, balance your blood-sugar levels, restore and stabilize your body's natural bioelectrical states, increase your energy, lower stress, relieve headaches, reduce or eliminate jet lag, accelerate healing, and protect your body against EMFs. As I write this, I'm grounded by a pink band on my wrist that's delivering the earth's recuperative energies to me.

## EQUINOX FITNESS

If you're near any of the clubs where Equinox has upscale, full-scale facilities (51 clubs at this writing, in New York, Chicago, Los Angeles, Florida, Boston, San Francisco, Dallas, and Washington, D.C.), I recommend that you join this temple to health that was voted "Best Gym in America" by *Fitness* magazine. When you take Zumba Fitness, Nia, Tabata, intenSati, Body Sculpt, Kettlebell Training, spinning, yoga, body conditioning, or other classes at Equinox Fitness, you'll be inspired to move, appreciate, tone, and respect your precious body—and have fun while doing it. If you join, tell the membership advisor that "Connie Sugar Shock Bennett" referred you.

## Hay House

It's my pleasure to recommend transformative books, CDs, DVDs, and card decks from this book's publisher, Hay House. You can find a host of great reads from the likes of such inspiring authors as Jerry and Esther Hicks, Jorge Cruise, Marianne Williamson, Caroline Myss, Tavis Smiley, Christiane Northrup, M.D., Wayne W. Dyer, Ph.D., and, of course, Louise Hay. You also can catch your favorite authors on Hay House Radio (www.hayhouseradio.com) and read empowering personal growth articles on www.HealYourLife.com. And you can attend transformative live events such as the *I Can Do It!* or *Movers & Shakers* conference, both of which wowed me. Get links to events I recommend at www.BeyondSugarShockFavorites.com.

## Institute for Integrative Nutrition (IIN): Health Coach Training

www.IntegrativeNutrition.com

If health and wellness interest you, then I recommend that you check out the Health Coach Program at the Institute for Integrative Nutrition. (I'm a 2006 graduate.) Founded in 1992, IIN is the world's largest nutrition education school, and it offers cutting-edge training in nutrition and wellness, as well as in valuable business skills. If you attend through its online training program, you'll get introduced to such intriguing concepts as bio-individuality, food energetics, and my favorite, "Primary Food." (This is an idea similar to my Sweetness Principle, but IIN founder Joshua Rosenthal and I arrived independently at our exciting concepts.) If you study at IIN, you'll also learn from many top experts, including Deepak Chopra, M.D.; Mark Hyman, M.D.; Andrew Weil, M.D.; and Geneen Roth. Since I'm an IIN graduate, people often contact me with questions about the school. To help you figure out if the program is a good fit for you, I've written a Sugar Shock Blog post to answer your Frequently Asked Questions. Just read it at http://tinyurl.com/IIN-Should-You-Go-Connie or do a search for IIN on my Sugar Shock Blog. If you call IIN, tell them that Connie Bennett, author of *Beyond Sugar Shock*, sent you.

## IT'S MORINGA

It's Moringa provides supplements, capsules, beverages, and beauty products derived from *Moringa Oleifera*, considered the most nutritious plant on earth, according to researcher Monica Marcu, Ph.D., author of *Miracle Tree.* Moringa reportedly contains more than 90 nutrients, 46 types of antioxidants, and 36 anti-inflammatories. Alleged claims include the plant's ability to enhance weight loss, curb sugar cravings, promote metabolism, support blood-sugar levels, boost your immune system, and improve sleep. What I like about this company—whose owner, Jude Ken-Kwofie, I met at a health conference where I spoke—is that at least 25 cents from each purchase is donated to improve nutrition and fight malnutrition via partnerships with such nonprofits as Vitamin Angels. Readers of this book get a 5 percent discount on purchases over $25.

## MIND MOVIES

In recent years, high-tech Mind Movies®—mini-films that you can easily create in a few minutes—have become popular with people worldwide, including Bob Proctor, Bob Doyle, John Assaraf, and others featured in *The Secret*. To create a Mind Movie, you simply take photos (your own or ones you find on the Internet), drag and drop them, and then add royalty-free music and affirmations (either prewritten or created by you). "What you're doing with a Mind Movie is tricking your brain into thinking, 'It's already happened,'" explains Natalie Ledwell, Mind Movies co-founder with her husband, Glen, and Ryan Higgins. "You're vibrationally matching those things you want to attract," adds Ledwell, who dropped from a size 14 to a size 10 with the help of a weight-loss Mind Movie she created.

## U.S. WELLNESS MEATS

If you're a meat eater, I urge you to check out U.S. Wellness Meats, which offers grass-fed beef from fifth-generation farmer John Wood. Research shows that a naturally occurring substance in beef, conjugated linoleic acid (CLA), reduces the incidence of cancer and suppresses growth of existing cancers in lab animals. Unlike regular beef, grass-fed beef contains an omega 6:3 ratio comparable to fish without the mercury. These meats contain no animal by-products; and animals are given *no* hormones, *no* irradiation, and *no* antibiotics. Check out their amazing beef jerky and beef sticks. They're the only ones I've been able to find online that are sugar-free.

## VibesUP!

www.vibesup.com/connie

VibesUP offers a variety of whimsical and practical products, which are made from live extracts of plants and natural crystals. You can get Earth-Nurtured Mats, reusable metal Earth Bottle water bottles, Divine Sole (grounding shoe inserts), Charging Coasters, toothpaste, and many other items designed to neutralize and release your toxic energy and reconnect you to Mother Nature's natural electrical energy. Before products are put on the market, founder/owner Kaitlyn Keyt—the winner of Eight Visionary Awards from the Coalition for Visionary Arts—consults with both a physicist and an energy practitioner, who test their frequencies on a bioresonance machine and measures how they affect human beings. As I write this, my water is sitting, getting energized by a round Earth-Nurtured Mat; I'm wearing my Earth Ionizer pendant; and I'm about to put on my Earth Nurtured Velcro Wraps before working out. Get a discount and special suggestions for readers of this book. Just say that Connie Bennett sent you.

## Vital Choice Wild Seafood & Organics

If you have sugar cravings, wild seafood rich in protein and healthy omega-3 fats can help satisfy your appetite. I invite you to check out Vital Choice, my favorite source for high-quality, nutritionally rich, sustainably harvested wild salmon and seafood, which is considered naturally low in mercury and other contaminants by the FDA and EPA. They also have great organic berries. All fish from Vital Choice— which is endorsed by many top doctors—is caught and flash-frozen within hours and shipped right to your doorstep. And it's incredibly yummy—unlike any sea-food you've ever had. I invite you to get my special Sugar Shock Freedom Foods Starter Pack, which includes: 1 Wild Salmon Sampler (six 6-ounce portions, including two portions each of Sockeye, Silver, and King Salmon); 1 Organic Berry Sampler (1 pound each of frozen organic blueberries, strawberries, raspberries, and blackberries—which are great to add to morning smoothies); 1 Organic Salmon/Seafood Marinade Mix (tasty and sugar-free, 2 ounces); 3 cans of Wild Red™ Traditional Sockeye (3.75 ounces each—easy to bring to work); and 6 Weil for Vital Choice™ Savory Country Style Salmon Sockeye Sausages. All products I selected contain no added sugars, nitrites, MSG, soy, corn, wheat, eggs, or dairy, and they are Kosher. You get a special discount since you're a reader of this book.

## X-ISER

Think you don't have time to work out? Just get an X-iser and join the sprint-training revolution. With science backing it up (as I told you earlier), you can get a full cardio workout in a few minutes a day and burst off fat and cravings, too. The X-iser is specifically designed for people of any age or fitness level to sprint-train. Come to think of it, my beloved X-iser is now beckoning me to start bursting. Beats sugar any old day!

## YOUNG LIVING ESSENTIAL OILS

You can use high-grade therapeutic essential oils to help combat your sugar cravings and balance your blood sugar, according to research. For instance, grapefruit may help lessen your sweet urges, dill may give you pancreatic support and lower your blood-glucose levels, and peppermint may suppress your appetite. Young Living Essential Oils is one of my favorite companies, because their oils—which you can use internally, topically, or through inhalation—use a "Seed to Seal" process, meaning their people grow the plants, cultivate, distill, produce, package, and deliver them straight to your doorstep. Move over, sugar! You'll find a new healthy way of getting high. Just take a whiff of some of my favorite soothing, invigorating, healing scents such as Valor, White Angelica, Peace & Calming, Peppermint, Thieves, and Pain Away.

**Disclosure:** These product suggestions and statements have not been evaluated by the Food and Drug Administration (FDA). These products are not intended to diagnose, treat, cure, or prevent any disease.

# CONNECT WITH US

## A Special Invitation from Your Sugar Freedom Coach Connie Bennett

Now that you've finished *Beyond Sugar Shock*, in some respects, we're near the end of our adventure together. But on a much deeper level, you're just getting started, because we're deepening our relationship. Well, that's my hope at least. Let's make your experience of this book the beginning of a long, sweeterlicious relationship, okay?

Please don't go it alone. There's no need. Reach out to us now—and often—for encouragement, inspiration, information, and compassion so we can continue our special, budding relationship. We're here to help you release your sugar addiction and bad habits, achieve a Mind-Body-Spirit balance, and Get a Life that Rocks.

Join us right now. No matter where you are on your journey or road to self-discovery and empowerment, we're waiting to give you a cyber-hug when you join our fast-growing movement.

### Get Free Goodies Galore

First of all, I'm committed to giving you lots of free stuff:

- **Facebook:** Join us on Facebook at www.Facebook.com/ SmartHabitsFans, where you can listen to Woo-Hoo, Feel-Good Theme Songs; read Smart Habits Tips; share gratitude thoughts; get links to interesting articles; find tasty, sugar-free recipes; learn about sugar research; and more. Just "Like" us and you're in. Then, get active.

- **Free Downloads:** Go to my website (www.BeyondSugarShock.com) to get transformational tapping, mindful eating, meditation, compassion, and Ho'oponopono audio programs, as well as recorded interviews with Happy, Successful Sugar Kickers.

- **Recommended Resources:** Get links to my favorite resources at www .BeyondSugarShock.com  or www.BeyondSugarShockFavorites.com.

- **Motivating Morsels E-zine:** Subscribe to my Motivating Morsels e-zine, which gives you helpful articles, tips, empowering tidbits, and other valuable updates.

- **Sugar Shock Blog:** Read and contribute thoughts to my provocative Sugar Shock Blog (www.SugarShockBlog.com), where I post my takes on research stories; share how-to articles, Sweet Sugar-Free Success Stories, tips to break free, sugar-free recipes, and my speaking schedule; give you links to Woo-Hoo, Feel-Good Theme Songs or weight-loss blogs; etc.

- *Gab with the Gurus Radio Show*: Find out about upcoming guests who will appear on my *Gab with the Gurus Radio Show*. Every week, I interview celebrities and best-selling authors in health, wealth, personal empowerment, social networking, the law of attraction, and relationships. Listen live Wednesdays at 2 P.M. EST or later at www .GabWithTheGurus.com or at www.Facebook.com/GabWithTheGurus. Or load segments for free on iTunes.

- **Join the Beyond Sugar Shock Freedom Community:** Become a member of the fast-growing, supportive Beyond Sugar Shock Freedom SparkTeam on SparkPeople.com. Join challenges; find Break-Free Buddies; get tips; and find or contribute sugar-free, gluten-free, dairy-free, and artificial-free recipes. Would you like to be a Community Leader? Let us know. Join us at http://teams.sparkpeople.com/ BeyondSugarShock, or just do a search for Beyond Sugar Shock.

- **YouTube:** Get entertained and intrigued at my YouTube channels. Get links on my website www.BeyondSugarShock.com.

- **Be in an Upcoming Book:** When you become a Sweet Success Story, share your tale and photos (before and after) at www.SugarShockBlog .com, and you may be chosen to be included in one of my next books. Also, share your recipes with us.

- **Twitter:** Follow me on Twitter at www.Twitter.com/SmartHabitsGirl.

- **HealYourLife.com:** Read articles and inspirational messages from me on this exciting website devoted to helping you thrive.

## Let Me Lead & Coach You to Freedom & Sweetness

I'm here to support, encourage, educate, and inspire you. In fact, I'd be honored to work closely with you to help you achieve your goals and dreams.

- **Join the Companion Course:** Sign up for the Beyond Sugar Shock companion program, The Sugar Freedom Now Course (or Break Free of Your Sugar Addiction in 6 Weeks Program) via teleseminars/ webinars, prerecorded programs, or a live event. See www .BreakFreeWithConnie.com.

- **Work Privately with Me:** Get a life-changing experience by working with me privately or in a group. Learn more at www .CoachingWithConnie.com.

- **Invite Me to Speak or Coach You:** Put together a group of at least 30 people, and I'll come to your area to speak or coach you. Invite me by clicking the Contact Connie button at www.BeyondSugarShock.com.

- **Health and Life Coaches:** Let me help you help your clients. Contact me for details.

- **Got a Cool Idea?** Let me know. I'm always seeking ways to serve you better.

Warmly, and with high hopes for your life-changing, Sweet Success,

Connie Bennett, CHHC, CPC, ACC,
Transformational Speaker & Sugar Freedom Coach

# BIBLIOGRAPHY

## INTRODUCTION FROM CONNIE BENNETT

Years before becoming a Sugar Freedom Coach, health coach, and life coach, I worked as a professional journalist (reporter, columnist, researcher, or editor) for a variety of newspapers, magazines, and websites.

In fact, often, I would grab one sugary or carb fix after another just to have the energy and concentration to get from one deadline to the next.

But soon after I quit sugar on doctor's orders in 1998 and personally experienced remarkable health benefits, including the disappearance of 44 of my ailments, I became journalistically driven to discover more about sugar's many dangers and to educate people around the world about my findings.

That led to my first book, *Sugar Shock!*, an exposé, which was released in 2007 and has been praised by many medical experts and best-selling authors, including Dr. Mehmet Oz, Dr. Christiane Northrup, and Marilu Henner.

*Sugar Shock!*, which became a bestseller, reveals how your sugar habit can lead to nearly 150 health hazards, such as heart disease, cancer, infertility, Alzheimer's disease, depression, hypoglycemia, premature wrinkles, early aging, and many other conditions. In the book, I cited scores of medical studies from the most prestigious, peer-reviewed medical journals, which supported my conclusions.

Likewise, I discovered more studies that show that when you quit or at least reduce your intake of sugar and refined carbs, you may be able to stop or reverse many medical conditions, have a better quality of life, and live longer.

While researching *Sugar Shock!*, it quickly became clear to me that just writing an exposé wasn't nearly enough. I needed to provide readers with an easy road map to help them replace sugar and toxic carbs with healthier foods and nourishing, non-food activities.

Now, *Beyond Sugar Shock,* the book you're holding in your hands and its six-week Mind-Body-Spirit program, reflect more than ten years of coaching, supporting, and educating sugar addicts around the world.

My research for *Beyond Sugar Shock* consisted of several different components. To begin, over the years, I've interviewed some 400 or more best-selling authors; transformational, Mind-Body-Spirit speakers and experts; cutting-edge physicians (most of whom received additional nutrition training); medical researchers; thought leaders; wellness practitioners; nutrition and fitness experts; food industry insiders and observers; and Law of Attraction visionaries.

You can listen to many interviews for this book on my *Gab with the Gurus Radio Show* (www.GabWithTheGurus.com) or in such paid teleseminar series as my Sugar Freedom Now Course, also called Break Free of Your Sugar Addiction in 6 Weeks Program (www.BreakFreeWithConnie.com), the Sweeter Holiday Summit (www .SweeterHoliday.com), and the Thrive, Don't Just Survive Program (www.Thrive-DontSurvive.com). Although interviews for this book were recorded, whenever citing experts, I later sent e-mails for their approval and verification.

Meanwhile, for more than a decade, with the help of part-time research assistants—all with impressive credentials—we evaluated hundreds of medical studies linking sugar and refined carbohydrates to various ailments and dangers. To our delight, at times, my research assistants—including the late health journalist and author Mary Kittel (1969–2004)—excitedly uncovered vital information that has received scant or little attention in the press.

Perhaps the most powerful method that I used to decide what to include in *Beyond Sugar Shock* came directly from my target audience, with whom I began connecting in August 2001 in various online communities.

Members of KickSugar, a Yahoo group I founded in November 2002, were particularly helpful. I created KickSugar, an international support group, to educate, inspire, encourage, and guide people with sugar issues, most of whom had weight challenges, a history of hypoglycemia, prediabetes, diabetes, or other medical ailments. Over the years, as KickSugar gained thousands of followers (and remained active for about five years), people began asking me the same questions over and over again.

In fact, then–Assistant Moderator Myra Pinkham and I kept track of the hundreds of questions. First, their valuable queries helped me realize what kinds of information, tools, and guidance sugar addicts need and seek.

Second, members' woes and concerns helped pave the way for my first quit-sugar program, which ultimately led, years later, to my current signature Sugar Freedom Now Course, and now, this book.

In 2005, when I began studying at the Institute for Integrative Nutrition (IIN) to become a certified holistic health coach, I began to work privately and in groups with sugar addicts. Next, I became a certified life coach with the Institute for Professional Excellence in Coaching (iPEC) to help my clients even more.

While working on *Beyond Sugar Shock,* I brought on (for the second time, as with *Sugar Shock!*), respected journalist, clinical dietitian, public educator, and certified wellness coach Gale Maleskey, M.S., R.D. The sharp, talented Maleskey has spent more than 15 years writing about healthy lifestyles, food and nutrition, alternative medicine, and medical consumerism. A former senior editor for *Prevention,* she also has authored or co-authored dozens of books, including *Nature's Medicines, The Hormone Connection,* and *Energy Forever.*

For additional support, I received assistance from health researchers/writers Carey Rossi, Sandra Gordon, Mark Fuerst, Rachel Martin, Beverly Burmeier, and Hollis Templeton.

Finally, to compile this bibliography, I assembled a team of qualified, thorough, and thoughtful young journalists, all of whom graduated from the undergraduate or graduate program at Northwestern University's prestigious Medill School of Journalism, which, incidentally, I also attended. Hilary Powell, Chris Gray, Jeremy Gordon, and Lana Birbrair all diligently fact-checked the information included below.

These researchers/reporters have bright futures ahead of them, and already they're getting praise and recognition from such leading media outlets as *The Oprah Winfrey Network, People, Fast Company,* and *Popular Science.*

What follows is a significant selection of many medical studies, articles, radio shows, and TV segments that were helpful to me as I wrote *Beyond Sugar Shock.* Whenever possible, I've included URLs, which were still current as I completed this book.

Also, please note that in Chapter 1, for "My S.A.D. to SWEET Story," when recounting incidents from the late 1990s with my friend Tracey (pseudonym), I had to take some dramatic license, because both my friend's and my memory were fuzzy on the details of this long-ago incident.

Adams, Claire et al. "Promoting Self-Compassionate Attitudes Toward Eating Among Restrictive and Guilty Eaters," *Journal of Social and Clinical Psychology* 26, no. 10 (2007): 1120–1144, https://webspace .utexas.edu/neffk/pubs/AdamsLearyeating%20attitudes.pdf (accessed September 28, 2011).

Adams, Mike. "The Real Reason Why Processed Meats Are So Dangerous to Your Health," NaturalNews .com (August 21, 2005): http://www.naturalnews.com/011148.html (accessed September 28, 2011).

Aitken, Sarah. "Is the Standard American Diet (SAD) Bad for Your Health?" *NaturalNews.com* (December 6, 2007): http://www.naturalnews.com/022331.html (accessed September 28, 2011).

Alderman, Lesley. "Using Hypnosis to Gain More Control Over Your Illness," *The New York Times* (April 15, 2011): http://www.nytimes.com/2011/04/16/health/16patient.html?ref=health (accessed September 28, 2011).

Alexander, Jane. "Get Fit Dancing: Dance to a Different Beat with Zumba: Latin America's Latest Dance Craze Is So Infectious You Won't Even Notice You're Exercising," *The Telegraph* (March 20, 2009): http://www.telegraph.co.uk/health/dietandfitness/5050441/Get-fit-dancing-Dance-to-a-different-beat -with-Zumba.html (accessed September 28, 2011).

Allen, James. *As a Man Thinketh*. New York: DeVorss & Company, 1948.

Alman, Brian. "Brian Alman on Finding Your Voice and Losing Weight," *Gab with the Gurus with Connie Bennett* (January 21, 2011): http://www.blogtalkradio.com/gabwiththegurus/2011/01/21/brian-alman -on-finding-your-voice-and-losing-weigh (accessed September 28, 2011).

———. "How to Find Your Voice & Keep Off Excess Weight in 2011," *Sweeter Holiday Summit with Connie Bennett* Session #37. Private program (Dec. 15, 2010): http://InstantTeleseminar .com/?eventid=16473711 (accessed September 30, 2011).

Al-Mosawi, Haider. "Two Simple Ways to Form New Habits Without Really Trying," *ZenHabits* (January 30, 2009): http://zenhabits.net/two-simple-ways-to-form-new-habits-without-really-trying/ (accessed September 28, 2011).

Altman, Donald. "Zumba: Party Hearty for the American Heart Association & Mindfulness Expert Donald Altman," *Gab with the Gurus Radio Show With Connie Bennett* (February 25, 2011): http://www.blog talkradio.com/gabwiththegurus/2011/02/25/zumba-party-hearty-for-the-american-heart-assocation -mindfulness-expert-donald-altman (accessed September 28, 2011).

American Diabetes Association. "Artificial Sweeteners," Diabetes.org: http://www.diabetes. org/food-and-fitness/food/what-can-i-eat/artificial-sweeteners/?utm_source=WWW&utm_ medium=FooterSlider4&utm_content=artificial-sweetener-feb2011&utm_campaign=CON (accessed September 28, 2011).

American Film Institute. "America's Funniest Movies: AFI's 100 Years, 1000 Laughs," *AFI.com:* http:// www.afi.com/Docs/100Years/laughs100.pdf (accessed September 28, 2011).

Anderson, J. et al. "Diet and Diabetes," *Colorado State University,* updated May 12, 2010: http://www .ext.colostate.edu/pubs/foodnut/09334.html (accessed September 28, 2011).

Ani. "Compassion Meditation: A Great Stress Buster," *The Times of India* (July 23, 2010): http://articles. timesofindia.indiatimes.com/2010-07-23/holistic-living/28298471_1_meditation-program-meditation -practices-compassion (accessed September 28, 2011).

# Bibliography

Apovian, Caroline. "Sugar-Sweetened Soft Drinks, Obesity, and Type 2 Diabetes." *The Journal of the American Medical Association* 292, no. 8 (2004): 978–979. doi: 10.1001/jama.292.8.978. http://jama .ama-assn.org/content/292/8/978.extract (accessed November 26, 2011).

Appleton, Nancy. "Can Sugar Kill You Slowly? Author Nancy Appleton Tells You How," *Gab with the Gurus with Connie Bennett*: http://www.blogtalkradio.com/gabwiththegurus/2009/10/20/can-sugar-kill -you-slowly-author-nancy-appleton-te (accessed October 15, 2011).

———. "Fructose Is No Answer for a Sweetener." http://articles.mercola.com/sites/articles /archive/2002/01/05/fructose-part-two.aspx (accessed November 20, 2011).

———. *Lick the Sugar Habit*. Garden City Park, NY: Avery Trade, 1988.

———. "*Lick the Sugar Habit*'s Dr. Nancy Appleton (addition to Great Worldwide Sugar-Out Challenge)," *Gab with the Gurus with Connie Bennett*: http://www.blogtalkradio.com/gabwith thegurus/2009/01/19/lick-the-sugar-habits-dr-nancy-appleton-addition-to-great-worldwide-sugar -outchallenge (accessed October 15, 2011).

———. "Sugar Can Kill You—Nancy Appleton Tells You How." *Gab with the Gurus with Connie Bennett*: http://www.blogtalkradio.com/gabwiththegurus/2010/04/14/sugar-can-kill-you--nancy-appleton-tells - you-how (accessed November 20, 2011).

———. Many interviews, phone conversations, and follow-up e-mails over 10 years.

Appleton, Nancy with G.N. Jacobs. "141 Reasons Sugar Ruins Your Health. (Just Kidding, It's 143)." http://nancyappleton.com/141-reasons-sugar-ruins-your-health/ (accessed November 20, 2011).

———. *Suicide by Sugar: A Startling Look at Our #1 National Addiction*. Garden City Park, NY: Square One Publishing, 2009.

Aronowitz, Abby. "Why You Can't Bowl Over Those Last 10 Pounds," *Diet.com* (August 15, 2008): http://www.diet.com/diet-solutions/index.php?scnm=Weight-Loss-Plateau&sc=7 (accessed September 28, 2011).

Assaraf, John. "John Assaraf from *The Secret*," *Gab with the Gurus with Connie Bennett* (September 9, 2010): http://www.blogtalkradio.com/gabwiththegurus/2010/09/09/johsn-assaraf-from-the-secret (accessed October 7, 2011).

Associated Press. "Are you a Flexitarian? Meat-Eating Vegetarians Transform the Movement." (March 16, 2004): http://www.msnbc.msn.com/id/4541605/ns/health-fitness/t/are-you-flexitarian/#.Tjra94LkaSo (accessed September 28, 2011).

Attwood, Janet. "Janet Attwood: How to Find Your Passion," *Gab with the Gurus with Connie Bennett* (February 15, 2011): http://www.blogtalkradio.com/gabwiththegurus/2011/02/15/janet-attwood-how -to-find-your-passion (accessed September 28, 2011).

Bachman, Katy. "Congress Gets Involved in Fight over Food Marketing Guidelines: New Voluntary Rules Have Been Tough Battle for Industry," *Adweek* (July 27, 2011): http://www.adweek.com/news /advertising-branding/congress-gets-involved-fight-over-food-marketing-guidelines-133694 (accessed September 28, 2011).

Baime, Michael et al. "Meditation: An Introduction," *National Center for Complementary and Alternative Medicine* (June 2010): http://nccam.nih.gov/health/meditation/overview.htm (accessed September 28, 2011).

Baron, K.G. et al. "Role of Sleep Timing in Caloric Intake and BMI," *Obesity (Silver Spring)* 19, no. 7 (July 2011): 1374–1381. http://www.ncbi.nlm.nih.gov/pubmed/21527892 (abstract accessed October 16, 2011).

Barrett, Julia. "Endocrine Disruptors: Estrogens in a Bottle?" *Environmental Health Perspectives* 117, no. A241 (June 2009): http://www.ncbi.nlm.nih.gov/pmc/articles/PMC2702426/ (accessed September 28, 2011).

Bennett, Connie. "12 Tips to Break Free of Your Sugar Addiction (FREE Audio Program) with Dr. Jacob Teitelbaum": http://www.sugarshockblog.com/get-12-tips-to-break-free-of-your-sugar-addiction-.html (accessed October 7, 2011).

———. "Before You Indulge This Holiday Season, Consider Nearly 150 Ways Sugar Ruins Your Health." http://www.sugarshockblog.com/2011/11/before-you-indulge-consider-146-ways-ways-sugar-ruins -your-health.html (accessed Nov. 20, 2011).

———. Break Free of Your Sugar Addiction in 6 Weeks Program (also called Sugar Freedom Now Course) with Jean Kristeller, Ph.D.; Jill Lane, C.N.C.; hypnotist Steve G. Jones; tapping guru Nick Ortner; and others. URLS not provided for this is a paid program, *www.BreakFreeWithConnie.com* (accessed October 7, 2011).

———. "Can You Go a Year Without Sugar? Join Blogger Dana Kennedy," *Sugar Shock! Blog* (April 9, 2010): http://www.sugarshockblog.com/2010/04/can-you-go-a-year-without-candy-join-blogger-dana -kennedy.html (accessed September 30, 2011).

———. "*The Dr. Oz Show*: The # 1 Food Dr. Oz Wants Out of Your House—Sugar," *Sugar Shock! Blog* (January 21, 2011): http://www.sugarshockblog.com/2011/01/the-1-food-dr-oz-wants-out-of-your -house-sugar.html (accessed October 1, 2011).

———. "Hypoglycemia: A Hidden Hell," excerpt from *Sugar Shock!*: http://www.authorviews.com /authors/bennett/obd.htm (accessed October 7, 2011).

———. "Is Sleep Deprivation Making You Suicidal?" *Huffington Post* (December 24, 2010): http://www .huffingtonpost.com/connie-bennett/take-your-meds-not-prescr_b_799499.html (accessed September 28, 2011).

———. "Jack LaLanne: In Loving Memory to the Fitness Guru and Anti-Sugar Pioneer" (January 25, 2011): http://www.huffingtonpost.com/connie-bennett/jack-lalanne-in-loving-me_b_813232.html (accessed September 28, 2011).

———. "Kick-Sugar Success Story: Felicia Desrosiers," *Sugar Shock! Blog* (November 19, 2006): http:// www.sugarshockblog.com/2006/11/kicksugar_succe.html (accessed September 30, 2011).

———. "Kick-Sugar Success Story: Jimmy Moore," *Sugar Shock! Blog* (September 10, 2006): http:// www.sugarshockblog.com/2006/09/kicksugar_succe_1.html (accessed September 28, 2011).

———. "Lyme Disease Featured on Dr. Mehmet Oz's *Oprah & Friends Radio Show*," *Sugar Shock! Blog* (December 1, 2008): http://www.sugarshockblog.com/2008/12/lyme-disease-featured-on-oprah -friends.html (accessed October 7, 2011).

# Bibliography

———. "Parenting: Seven Simple Steps to a Sweeter You," (May 7, 2010): http://www.drlaura.com/b /Seven-Simple-Steps-to-a-Sweeter-You--/8568.html (accessed October 7, 2011).

———. "Sugar Hits the News, Thanks to Dr. Lustig's YouTube Video and Nightline," Video. *Huffington Post.com* (March 19, 2010): http://www.huffingtonpost.com/connie-bennett/sugar-hits-the-news -thank_b_506517.html (accessed November 23, 2011).

———. *Sweeter Holiday Summit 2010.* Teleseminar series, paid, that features interviews with 38 experts in health, wellness, personal empowerment, the law of attraction, meditation, relationships, and more: http://www.sweeterholiday.com/ (accessed October 7, 2011).

———. *Thrive, Don't Just Survive.* Teleseminar series that features interviews with 12 top health and wellness experts. Jan–March 2009: *www.ThriveDontSurvive.com* (accessed October 7, 2011).

Bennett, Connie and Stephen Sinatra. *Sugar Shock! How Sweets and Simple Carbs Can Derail Your Life— And How You Can Get Back on Track.* New York: Berkley Publishing Group, 2007.

Berkey, C.S. et al. "Sugar-Added Beverages and Adolescent Weight Change." *Obesity Research* 12 (2004): 7678–788. http://www.ncbi.nlm.nih.gov/pubmed/15166298 (abstract accessed October 1, 2011).

Beyond Sugar Shock Freedom SparkTeam: http://www.sparkpeople.com/myspark/groups_individual .asp?gid=51006 (accessed October 7, 2011).

Bilger, Burkhard. "The Search for Sweet: Building a Better Sugar Substitute." *The New Yorker* 14 (May 22, 2006): 40. http://www.newyorker.com/archive/2006/05/22/060522fa_fact_bilger (abstract accessed November 30, 2011).

Bittman, Mark. "Bad Food? Tax It, and Subsidize Vegetables," *The New York Times* (July 23, 2011): http://www.nytimes.com/2011/07/24/opinion/sunday/24bittman.html?_r=1 (accessed September 28, 2011).

———. "Can Big Food Regulate Itself? Fat Chance." *The New York Times* (August 2, 2011): http:// opinionator.blogs.nytimes.com/2011/08/02/when-big-food-makes-its-own-rules/ (accessed September 28, 2011).

———. "Junk Food 'Guidelines' Won't Help," *The New York Times* (May 3, 2011): http://opinionator .blogs.nytimes.com/2011/05/03/junk-food-guidelines-wont-help/ (accessed September 28, 2011).

Biziou, Barbara. "Rituals to Have a Happy New Year & to Lose Weight with Barbara Biziou," *Gab with the Gurus with Connie Bennett* (January 11, 2011): http://www.blogtalkradio.com/gabwiththegu rus/2011/01/11/rituals-to-have-a-happy-new-year-to-lose-weight-with-barbara-biziou (accessed October 16, 2011).

Bloch, Douglas. *Words That Heal: Affirmations and Meditations for Daily Living.* Portland, OR: Pallas Communications, 1998.

Block, Gladys. "Foods Contributing to Energy Intake in the US: Data from NHANES III and NHANES 1999–2000." *Journal of Food Composition and Analysis* 17 (June–August 2004): 439–447. http://www .sciencedirect.com/science/article/pii/S0889157504000328 (abstract accessed October 16, 2011).

Block, Keith. Interview and follow-up e-mails with the cancer specialist and author.

Bohn, Torsten et al. "Phytic Acid Added to White-Wheat Bread Inhibits Fractional Apparent Magnesium Absorption in Humans," *American Journal of Clinical Nutrition* 79: (March 2004): 418–423. http://www.ajcn.org/content/79/3/418 (abstract accessed September 28, 2011).

Bouchez, Colette. "The Dream Diet: Losing Weight While You Sleep," *WebMD* (January 1, 2007): http://www.webmd.com/sleep-disorders/guide/lose-weight-while-sleeping?page=2 (accessed September 28, 2011).

———. "Yoga for Weight Loss?" Medicine.net (July 21, 2006): http://www.medicinenet.com/script/main/art.asp?articlekey=63034 (accessed September 28, 2011).

Bowden, Jonny. *The 150 Most Effective Ways to Boost Your Energy: The Surprising, Unbiased Truth about Using Nutrition, Exercise, Supplements, Stress Relief, and Personal Empowerment to Stay Energized All Day.* Beverly, MA: Fair Winds Press, 2008.

———. Phone conversations and e-mails about protein requirements.

Boyles, Salynn. "Low-Carb Diets Improve Cholesterol Long Term," *WebMD*: http://www.webmd.com/cholesterol-management/news/20100802/low-carb-diets-improve-cholesterol-long-term (accessed October 16, 2011).

Brady, Elizabeth. "Kevin Smith and Others Shamed into Losing Weight by an Airline," *AOL Travel* (February 10, 2011): http://news.travel.aol.com/2011/02/10/kevin-smith-and-others-shamed-into-losing-weight-by-an-airline/ (accessed September 28, 2011).

Brahm, Ajahn. "Metta to the Present," JustBeGood.net (May 14, 2008): http://www.justbegood.net/Downloads/Ajarn%20Brahm%27s%20Talks%203/Metta%20to%20the%20Present.MP3 (accessed September 28, 2011).

Bray, G.A. et al. "Consumption of High-Fructose Corn Syrup in Beverages May Play a Role in the Epidemic of Obesity," *American Journal of Clinical Nutrition* 79 (2004): 537–543. http://www.ajcn.org/content/79/4/537.full.pdf+html (accessed October 1, 2011).

Breus, Michael. *"Gab with Gurus* Turns 3: Lauren E. Miller & Dr. Michael Breus," *Gab with the Gurus with Connie Bennett* (June 13, 2011): http://www.blogtalkradio.com/gabwiththegurus/2011/06/13/gab-with-gurus-turns-3-lauren-e-miller-dr-michael-breus (accessed October 16, 2011).

———. *The Sleep Doctor's Diet Plan: Lose Weight Through Better Sleep.* United States: Rodale Books, 2011.

Brown, Kyle. "SAD (Standard American Diet) Makes No Sense," Video. The Cardiovascular Disease Foundation's speaker, Nutritionist Kyle Brown discusses healthy eating habits at Rancho Carlsbad Senior Community (October 22, 2009): http://www.youtube.com/watch?v=vzEU0KG7Lfl (accessed September 28, 2011).

Buddharakkhita, Acharya. "Metta: The Philosophy and Practice of Universal Love," *Access to Insight*: http://www.accesstoinsight.org/lib/authors/buddharakkhita/wheel365.html (accessed September 28, 2011).

Burros, Marian. "Now What? U.S. Study Says Margarine May Be Harmful," *The New York Times* (October 7, 1992): http://www.nytimes.com/1992/10/07/garden/now-what-us-study-says-margarine-may-be-harmful.html?pagewanted=all&src=pm (accessed October, 16, 2011).

# Bibliography

Bushman, Tavaner. "Mood-Boosting Foods," *Chicago Sun-Times* (February 15, 2011): http://www.sun times.com/lifestyles/food/3776799-423/mood-boosting-foods.html (accessed September 28, 2011).

Byrne, Rhonda. *The Secret*. New York: Atria, 2006.

Campaign for a Commercial-Free Childhood. Letter from Susan Linn, EdD and Alvin F. Poussaint, M.D.

————. Letter from Susan Linn on behalf of the CCFC Steering Committee to Mr. Jon Leibowitz, Chairman of the Federal Trade Commission (June 24, 2009): http://www.commercialfreechildhood.org/pdf /lettertoftcjune09.pdf (accessed October 6, 2011).

Cashmore, Pete. "Southwest Tweets, Blogs Apology to Kevin Smith," Mashable.com (February 14, 2010): http://mashable.com/2010/02/14/southwest-kevin-smith/ (accessed September 28, 2011).

CeliacCentral.org. "The Gluten-Free Diet": http://www.celiaccentral.org/SiteData/docs/The%20 gluten/13ec19c2616ddac0/The%20gluten%20free%20diet.pdf (accessed October 16, 2011).

Center for Science in the Public Interest. "Chemical Cuisine," Cspinet.org: http://www.cspinet.org /reports/chemcuisine.htm (accessed November 23, 2011).

————. "CSPI's Petition to the FDA to Require Better Sugar Labeling on Foods": http://www.cspinet .org/reports/sugar/sugarpet1.pdf (accessed October 16, 2011).

————. "Dieting Figures—Trends and Statistics," CSPInet.org: http://www.cspinet.org/new/201004141 .html (accessed September 28, 2011).

————. "Health Advocates Cheer Decline in Soda Drinking" (April 14, 2010): http://www.cspinet.org /new/201004141.html (accessed September 28, 2011).

Centers for Disease Control and Prevention. "Successes and Opportunities for Population-Based Prevention and Control at a Glance 2011," cdc.gov (August 1, 2011): http://www.cdc.gov/chronicdisease /resources/publications/AAG/ddt.htm (accessed November 23, 2011).

Chan, Amanda. "Warding Off Depression: 'Mindfulness' Therapy Works as Well as Drugs," *My Health News Daily* (December 6, 2010): http://www.myhealthnewsdaily.com/being-mindful-of-emotions -could-prevent-depression-relapse-as-well-as-drugs-0836/ (accessed September 28, 2011).

Chapelot, Didier and Jeanine Louis-Sylvestre. "Relevance of Energy Expenditure and Energy Intake to the Etiology of Obesity," *The American Journal of Clinical Nutrition* 76 (August 2002): 489. http://www.ajcn .org/content/76/2/489.1.full.pdf+html (accessed October 16, 2011).

Chen, L. "Reduction in Consumption of Sugar-Sweetened Beverages Is Associated with Weight Loss: The Premier Trial." http://www.ncbi.nlm.nih.gov/pubmed/19339405 (accessed Nov. 26, 2011).

Chen, Mei-Yen and Jenny C. Liao. "Relationship Between Attendance at Breakfast and School Achievement among Nursing Students," *Journal of Nursing Research* 10: (March 2002): http://journals.lww .com/jnr-twna/Abstract/2002/03000/Relationship_Between_Attendance_at_Breakfast_and.2.aspx (abstract accessed September 28, 2011).

Cherniack, E.P. "Potential Applications for Alternative Medicine to Treat Obesity in an Aging Population," *Alternative Medicine Review* 13: (2008): 34–42. http://www.ncbi.nlm.nih.gov/pubmed/18377101 (accessed September 28, 2011).

Cheung, Lilian. "Dr. Lilian Cheung on Mindful Eating," *Gab with the Gurus with Connie Bennett* (March 18, 2011): http://www.blogtalkradio.com/gabwiththegurus/2011/03/18/lilian-cheung-on-mindful -eating (accessed September 28, 2011).

Coconut Research Center. "Coconut": http://www.coconutresearchcenter.org/ (accessed September 28, 2011).

Colditz, Graham A. et al. "The Nurses' Health Study: 20-Year Contribution to the Understanding of Health among Women," *Journal of Women's Health* 6 (February 1997): 49–62. http://www.ncbi.nlm.nih .gov/pubmed/9065374?dopt=Abstract (abstract accessed October 16, 2011).

Conley, Mikaela. "'Caveman Diet' Gets Modern Day Support," *ABC News* (June 22, 2011): http://abc news.go.com/Health/caveman-diet-online-support/story?id=13897179 (accessed September 28, 2011).

Cooper, Ann. "Ann Cooper Talks School Lunches," Video. Ted.com. December 2007. http://www.ted .com/talks/lang/en/ann_cooper_talks_school_lunches.html (accessed November 30, 2011).

Cordain, Loren. "Cereal Grains: Humanity's Double-Edged Sword," *World Review of Nutrition and Dietetics* 84 (1999): 19–73. http://thepaleodiet.com/wp-content/uploads/2011/02/Cerealgrainhumanitydou blesword.pdf (accessed September 28, 2011).

———. *The Paleo Diet: Lose Weight and Get Healthy by Eating the Food You Were Designed to Eat.* Hoboken, New Jersey: John Wiley & Sons, 2002.

Cousins, Norman. *Anatomy of an Illness as Perceived by the Patient.* New York: Bantam Books, 1991.

———. "Conversations with History: Norman Cousins," Video. http://www.youtube.com/watch?v=oas -WpnpQpk (accessed October 17, 2011).

Craig, Gary. EFT (Emotional Freedom Techniques®): http://www.emofree.com/ (accessed October 16, 2011).

Cuffey, Abigail. "8 Amazing Blogger Weight-Loss Transformations," *Woman's Day* (January 6, 2011): http://health.yahoo.net/articles/weight-loss/8-amazing-blogger-weight-loss-transformations (accessed September 28, 2011).

Dangour, Alan D. et al. "Nutritional Quality of Organic Foods: A Systematic Review," *American Journal of Clinical Nutrition* (July 29, 2009): http://ag.utah.gov/learn/documents/organicnutritionstudy.pdf (accessed September 28, 2011).

Dasilva, Sergio G. et al. "Psychophysiological Responses to Self-Paced Treadmill and Overground Exercise," *Medicine & Science in Sports & Exercise* 43 (June 2011): 1114–1124. http://journals.lww.com /acsm-msse/Abstract/2011/06000/Psychophysiological_Responses_to_Self_Paced.26.aspx (accessed September 28, 2011).

DeNoon, Daniel J. "7 Rules for Eating: Choose Food Over Food-Like Substances, Food Writer Michael Pollan Tells CDC," *WebMD Health News* (March 23, 2009): http://www.webmd.com/food-recipes /news/20090323/7-rules-for-eating (accessed September 28, 2011).

Desrosiers, Felicia. E-mail correspondence for "Sweet Success Story: How Being Sugar-Free Makes Me Happy, Creative & Symptom-Free."

Dolson, Laura. "Fructose: Sweet, But Dangerous," *About.com* (October 9, 2008): http://lowcarbdiets .about.com/od/nutrition/a/fructosedangers.htm (accessed September 28, 2011).

Dona A., and I.S. Arvanitoyannis. "Health Risks of Genetically Modified Foods," *Critical Reviews in Food, Science, and Nutrition* 49, no. 2 (February 2009):164–175. Department of Forensic Medicine and Toxicology, University of Athens, Medical School, Athens, Greece. http://www.ncbi.nlm.nih.gov /pubmed/18989835 (abstract accessed September 30, 2011).

Donovan, Travis Walter. "9 Most Misleading Food Labels," *Huffington Post* (June 20, 2010): http://www .huffingtonpost.com/2010/04/20/9-most-misleading-food-la_n_538868.html#s81059&title=All_Natural (accessed September 28, 2011).

Downie, Chris. "SparkPeople's Chris Downie & K.C. Craichy on The Super Health Diet," *Gab with the Gurus with Connie Bennett* (February 17, 2011): http://www.blogtalkradio.com/gabwiththe gu rus/2011/02/17/sparkpeoples-chris-downie-kc-craichy-on-the-super-health-diet (accessed October 16, 2011).

*Dr. Oz Show, The.* "Mediation Techniques Demonstrated by Deepak Chopra," Video. http://www.doctor oz.com/videos/deepak-chopra-meditation (accessed September 28, 2011).

———. "The # 1 Food You Need to Lose": http://www.doctoroz.com/videos/1-food-you-need-lose -pt-1; http://www.doctoroz.com/videos/1-food-you-need-lose-pt-2; and http://www.doctoroz.com /videos/1-food-you-need-lose-pt-3 (accessed October 1, 2011).

———. "Cutting-Edge Cravings Killers," Video. http://www.doctoroz.com/videos/cutting-edge -cravings-killers (accessed October 1, 2011).

Druck, Ken. "How to Cope Well with Life's Losses Over the Holidays," *Sweeter Holiday Summit with Connie Bennett* Session #20 (December 7, 2010): http://InstantTeleseminar.com/?eventid=16232043 (accessed September 30, 2011).

Dufty, William. *Sugar Blues.* New York: Warner Books, 1986.

Dwoskin, Hale. "Hale Dwoskin on The Sedona Method," *Gab with the Gurus with Connie Bennett* (January 18, 2011): http://www.blogtalkradio.com/gabwiththegurus/2011/01/18/hale-dwoskin-on-the -sedona-method (accessed September 28, 2011).

———. *The Sedona Method: Your Key to Lasting Happiness, Success, Peace, and Emotional Well-Being.* Sedona, AZ: Sedona Press, 2003.

Dyer, Wayne W. *The Power of Intention: Learning to Co-create Your World Your Way.* Carlsbad, CA: Hay House, 2005.

———. *There's a Spiritual Solution to Every Problem.* New York: Quill, 2003.

Eades, Michael and Mary Dan Eades. *The 30-Day Low-Carb Diet Solution.* Hoboken, New Jersey: John Wiley & Sons, 2003.

Eating Addictions Anonymous. "The SANE Fellowship": http://dcregistry.com/users/eatingaddictions/ (accessed September 28, 2011).

Edlund, Matthew. *The Power of Rest: Why Sleep Alone Is Not Enough. A 30-Day Plan to Reset Your Body.* New York: HarperOne, 2011.

Elliott, Debbie. "At End-of-the-Line Prison, An Unlikely Escape," *NPR.org* (February 8, 2011): http://www.npr.org/2011/02/08/133505880/at-end-of-the-line-prison-an-unlikely-escape (accessed September 30, 2011).

Elliott, Sharon et al. "Fructose, Weight Gain, and the Insulin Resistance Syndrome" http://www.ajcn.org/content/76/5/911.full?sid=67e7d2c5-15ad-41a4-ad49-8426cc85d462 (accessed November 20, 2011).

Emmons, Robert. *Thanks! How Practicing Gratitude Can Make You Happier.* United States: Mariner Books, 2008.

Emmons, Robert and Michael E. McCullough. "Counting Blessings Versus Burdens: An Experimental Investigation of Gratitude and Subjective Well-Being in Daily Life," *Journal of Personality and Social Psychology* 84, no. 2 (2003): 377–389. http://www.chucklin.org/wp-content/uploads/2010/02/Emmons_McCullough_2003_JPSP.pdf (accessed October 16, 2011).

———. "Highlights from the Research Project on Gratitude and Thankfulness," *University of Miami* (2003): http://www.psy.miami.edu/faculty/mmccullough/Gratitude-Related%20Stuff/highlights_fall_2003.pdf (accessed October 16, 2011).

Emory University. "MedicalHorizon: Added Sugars Increase Heart Disease Risk Factors," Video. http://www.youtube.com/watch?v=MPTTsltWfX8 (accessed October 15, 2011).

Emory Woodruff Health Sciences Center. "Higher Amounts of Added Sugars Increase Heart Disease Risk Factors": http://shared.web.emory.edu/whsc/news/releases/2010/04/higher-amounts-of-added-sugars-increase-heart-disease-risk-factors.html (accessed October 1, 2011).

EngineeringToolBox.com "Unit Converter with the Most Common Units": http://www.engineeringtoolbox.com/unit-converter-d_185.html#Mass (accessed October 16, 2011).

Environmental Working Group. "Executive Summary": http://www.ewg.org/foodnews/summary/ (accessed September 28, 2011).

———. "The Full List: 53 Fruits and Vegetables": http://www.ewg.org/foodnews/list (accessed September 28, 2011).

Epley, Richard J. et al. "Nitrite in Meat," *University of Minnesota* (1992): http://www.extension.umn.edu/distribution/nutrition/DJ0974.html (accessed September 28, 2011).

European Commission, Scientific Committee on Food. "New Findings Regarding the Presence of Acrylamide in Food: Health & Consumer Protection Directorate-General" (July 3, 2002): http://ec.europa.eu/food/fs/sc/scf/out131_en.pdf (accessed September 30, 2011).

Evert, Alison. "Caffeine in the Diet," *Medline Plus* (May 5, 2011): http://www.nlm.nih.gov/medlineplus/ency/article/002445.htm (accessed September 28, 2011).

*Extreme Makeover: Home Edition.* "Guinta Family," Video. (May 11, 2008): http://www.youtube.com/watch?v=6wneBut3gok (accessed October 16, 2011).

Facebook. Smart Habits Fans, fan page for Connie Bennett, www.Facebook.com/SmartHabitsFans. Also see www.Facebook.com/BeyondSugarShock, www.Facebook.com/GabWithTheGurus (accessed October 7, 2011).

Fain, Jean. "Self-Compassion to Lose Weight with Jean Fain," *Gab with the Gurus with Connie Bennett* (March 14, 2011): http://www.blogtalkradio.com/gabwiththegurus/2011/03/14/self-compassion-to -lose-weight-with-jean-fain (accessed September 28, 2011).

———. "Self-Compassion: Kiss Your Inner Drill Sergeant Goodbye," *Huffington Post* (February 8, 2011): http://www.huffingtonpost.com/jean-fain-licsw-msw/self-compassion_b_819808.html (accessed September 28, 2011).

———. *The Self-Compassion Diet: A Step-by-Step Program to Lose Weight with Loving-Kindness.* Boulder, CO: Sounds True, 2010.

Flegg, Anita. *Hypoglycemia: The Other Sugar Disease.* United States: Book Coach Press, 2006.

Ford, Arielle. "Arielle Ford: Manifest Your Soulmate," *Gab with the Gurus with Connie Bennett* (January 26, 2011): http://www.blogtalkradio.com/gabwiththegurus/2011/01/26/arielle-ford-manifest-your -soulmate (accessed September 28, 2011).

Forgione, Mary. "What is Natural About Natural Food?" *Los Angeles Times* (October 1, 2010): http:// articles.latimes.com/2010/oct/01/news/la-heb-benandjerry-20101001 (accessed September 28, 2011).

Friedman, Philip H. "Forgiveness is the Solution with Dr. Philip Friedman." *Gab with the Gurus with Connie Bennett* (August 9, 2010): http://www.blogtalkradio.com/gabwiththegurus/2010/08/09/forgiveness -is-the-solution-with-dr-philip-friedma (accessed October 16, 2011).

———. *The Forgiveness Solution: The Whole-Body Rx for Finding True Happiness, Abundant Love, and Inner Peace.* San Francisco: Conari Press, 2010.

Gaiam.com. "A Quote by Jon Kabat-Zinn on non-doing, courage, stillness, activity, and purpose," Gaiam Life: http://blog.gaiam.com/quotes/authors/jon-kabat-zinn (accessed September 30, 2011).

Gans, Keri. "Keri Gans and 'The Small Change Diet,'" *Gab with the Gurus with Connie Bennett* (March 24, 2011): http://www.blogtalkradio.com/gabwiththegurus/2011/03/24/keri-gans-and-the-small-change -diet (accessed September 28, 2011).

Garcia, Oz and Sharyn Kolberg. *Look and Feel Fabulous Forever: The World's Best Supplements, Anti-Aging Techniques, and High-Tech.* New York: HarperCollins, 2002.

Gearhardt, Ashley N. et al. "Food Addiction: An Examination of the Diagnostic Criteria for Dependence," *Journal of Addiction Medicine* 3, no. 1 (March 2009): 1–7. http://journals.lww.com/journal addictionmedicine/Abstract/2009/03000/Food_Addiction__An_Examination_of_the_Diagnostic.1.aspx (accessed November 23, 2011).

Gerbarg, Patricia L. and Richard P. Brown. "Yoga: A Breath of Relief for Hurricane Katrina Refugees," *Current Psychiatry* 4, no. 10 (October 2005): 55–67. http://www.currentpsychiatry.com/pdf/0410/0410CP _Article3.pdf (accessed September 28, 2011).

Germer, Christopher. "Meditations: Downloads." MindfulSelfCompassion.org: http://www.mindfulself compassion.org/meditations_downloads.php (accessed September 28, 2011).

Gershoff, S.N. "Nutrition Evaluation of Dietary Fat Substitutes," *Nutrition Reviews* 53, no. 11 (November 1995): 305–313. http://www.ncbi.nlm.nih.gov/sites/entrez?Db=pubmed&Cmd=Retrieve& list_uids=8643212&dopt=abstractplus (accessed October 16, 2011).

Ghirardelli Chocolate Company. "About Ghirardelli Chocolate: Frequently Asked Questions": http://www.ghirardelli.com/about/faq_chocolate.aspx (accessed September 28, 2011).

GI Diet Guide, The. "The GI Diet—List of Low GI Foods": http://www.the-gi-diet.org/lowgifoods/ (accessed September 28, 2011).

Giovannucci, Edward L. "Obesity, Insulin Resistance, and Cancer Risk," *Cancer Prevention, The New York-Presbyterian Hospital* (Spring 2005): http://www.nypcancerprevention.com/issue/5/pro/pro_features/pre_ear.shtml (accessed September 28, 2011).

Gittleman, Ann Louise. *Fat Flush for Life: The Year-Round Super Detox Plan to Boost Your Metabolism and Keep the Weight Off Permanently*. Philadelphia: Da Capo Lifelong Books, 2011.

———. *The Fat Flush Plan*. United States: McGraw-Hill, 2002.

———. *Get the Sugar Out: 501 Simple Ways to Cut the Sugar Out of Any Diet*. New York: Three Rivers Press, 1996. 2 Rev Upd edition (January 8, 2008).

———. "Lose Weight for Life with Ann Louise Gittleman," *Gab with the Gurus with Connie Bennett* (Aug. 31, 2011): http://www.blogtalkradio.com/gabwiththegurus/2011/08/31/lose-weight-for-life-with-ann-louise-gittleman (accessed September 30, 2011).

———. *Zapped: Why Your Cell Phone Shouldn't Be Your Alarm Clock and 1,268 Ways to Outsmart the Hazards of Electronic Pollution*. New York: HarperOne, 2010.

Glass, Kellie. "Eating Healthy vs. Standard American Diet," *Livestrong* (March 28, 2011): http://www.livestrong.com/article/409750-eating-healthy-vs-standard-american-diet/ (accessed September 28, 2011).

Glueck, Charles J. et al. "Dietary Fat Substitutes," *Nutrition Research* 14, no. 10 (October 1994): 1605–1619. http://www.sciencedirect.com/science/article/pii/S0271531705802398 (accessed October 16, 2011).

Goldstone, A.P. et al. "Fasting Biases Brain Reward Systems Towards High-Calorie Foods," *European Journal of Neuroscience* 30, no. 8 (October 2009): 1625–1635. http://www.ncbi.nlm.nih.gov/pubmed/19811532 (abstract accessed September 28, 2011).

*Good Morning America*. "Do You Need a Health Coach? An Interview with Dr. Edward Phillips," Video. (January 6, 2010): http://abcnews.go.com/video/playerIndex?id=9493792 (accessed September 28, 2011).

———. "New Year, New You: Dr. Oz's Tips to Lose Weight," Video. http://abcnews.go.com/GMA/video/new-year-new-you-dr-ozs-tips-to-lose-weight-12580996 (accessed September 30, 2011).

Goodreads. "Hippocrates Quotes": http://www.goodreads.com/author/quotes/248774.Hippocrates_000100_7.htm (accessed September 28, 2011).

Gould, Roger. "Get Help to End Emotional Eating with Dr. Roger Gould," *Gab with the Gurus with Connie Bennett* (October 6, 2010): http://www.blogtalkradio.com/gabwiththegurus/2010/10/06/get-help-to-end-emotional-eating-with-dr-roger-gould (accessed September 28, 2011).

Graybiel, A.M. "Habits, Rituals, and the Evaluative Brain," *Annual Review of Neuroscience* 31 (2008): 359–387. http://www.ncbi.nlm.nih.gov/pubmed/18558860 (abstract accessed September 28, 2011).

# Bibliography

Greeson, Jeffrey M. "Mindfulness Research Update: 2008," *Journal of Evidence-Based Complementary & Alternative Medicine* 14, no. 1 (January 2009): 10–18. http://chp.sagepub.com/content/14/1/10 (abstract accessed September 28, 2011).

Grocery Manufacturers Association. "About Acrylamide": http://www.acrylamidefacts.org/About%20 Acrylamide.aspx (accessed October 15, 2011).

Grogan, Martha. "Does the Sodium Nitrate in Processed Meat Increase my Risk of Heart Disease?" *Mayo Clinic* (November 11, 2010): http://www.mayoclinic.com/health/sodium-nitrate/AN02119 (accessed September 28, 2011).

Grossman, Paul et al. "Mindfulness-Based Stress Reduction and Health Benefits: A Meta-Analysis," *Journal of Psychosomatic Research* 57, no. 1 (July 2004): 35–43. http://www.epilepsiezentrum .uniklinik-freiburg.de/medmed/live/literatur/MBSR_MA_JPR_2004.pdf (accessed September 28, 2011).

Grotto, David and Elisa Zied. "The Standard American Diet and its Relationship to the Health Status of Americans," *Nutrition in Clinical Practice* 25, no. 6 (December 2010): 603–612. http://ncp.sagepub .com/content/25/6/603.full (accessed September 28, 2011).

Hahn II., James. Phone calls and e-mail follow-ups for "James Hahn II's Sweet Success Story: How Lent Inspired Me to Quit Sugar as Penance & Lose 87 Pounds."

Haley, Stephen. "Sugar and Sweeteners Outlook," United States Department of Agriculture (May 16, 2011): http://www.ers.usda.gov/publications/sss/2011/05May/SSSM273.pdf (accessed November 20, 2011).

Hamilton-Romeo, Réal. "Sleep and Lose—Weight, That Is," *Gab with the Gurus with Connie Bennett* (February 22, 2011): http://www.blogtalkradio.com/gabwiththegurus/2011/02/22/sleep-and-lose--weight -that-is (accessed September 30, 2011).

Harp, David. "Become a 3-Minute Meditator," *Gab with the Gurus with Connie Bennett* (March 17, 2011): http://www.blogtalkradio.com/gabwiththegurus/2011/03/17/david-harp-become-a-three -minute-meditator (accessed October 16, 2011).

Harp, David and Nana Smiley. *The Three Minute Mediator: Reduce Stress. Control Fear. Diminish Anger. In Almost No Time At All. Anywhere. Anytime.* United States: Mind's I Press, 2008.

Harvard Health Publications. "Glycemic Index and Glycemic Load For 100+ Foods": http://www.health .harvard.edu/newsweek/Glycemic_index_and_glycemic_load_for_100_foods.htm (accessed September 28, 2011).

Hawkes, Corinna. "Marketing Food to Children: Changes in the Global Regulatory Environment 2004– 2006." http://whqlibdoc.who.int/publications/2007/9789240682122_eng.pdf

Hay, Louise L. *Heal Your Body A-Z: The Mental Causes for Physical Illness and the Way to Overcome Them.* Carlsbad, CA: Hay House, 1998.

———. *I Can Do It: How to Use Affirmations to Change Your Life.* Affirmation CD. Carlsbad, CA: Hay House, 2004.

———. *Stress Free: Peaceful Affirmations to Relieve Anxiety and Help you Relax.* Audiobook and CD. Carlsbad, CA: Hay House, 2004.

————. *You Can Heal Your Life*. Carlsbad, CA: Hay House, 2009.

Hayashi, Keiko et al. "Laughter Lowered the Increase in Postprandial Blood Glucose," *Diabetes Care* 26, no. 5 (May 2003): 1651–1652. http://care.diabetesjournals.org/content/26/5/1651.full.pdf+htm (accessed September 28, 2011).

Hellmich, Nanci. "Sleep-Deprived People Eat 300 More Calories a Day," *USA Today* (March 23, 2011): http://yourlife.usatoday.com/health/story/2011/03/Sleep-deprived-people-eat-300-more-calories-a -day/45227686/1?sms_ss=twitter&at_xt=4d8b76a9d07e3f6a%2C0 (accessed September 28, 2011).

Hendrick, Bill. "Many Sleep-Deprived Americans Blame Stress," *WebMD:* http://www.webmd.com /sleep-disorders/news/20101111/many-sleep-deprived-americans-blame-stress (accessed November 29, 2011).

Hill, Napoleon. "Napoleon Hill—What the Mind Can Conceive, Believe & Achieve," Video. http://www .youtube.com/watch?v=2hA-7aq6OXI  (accessed November 29, 2011).

————. *Think and Grow Rich*. Rockville: Arc Manor, 2007, and New York: Ballantine Books, 1987.

Hobson, Katherine. "Can Snacks be Part of a Healthful Diet?" *U.S. News & World Report* (June 18, 2009): http://health.usnews.com/health-news/diet-fitness/articles/2009/06/18/can-snacks-be-part-of-a-health ful-diet?s_cid=related-links:TOP (accessed September 28, 2011).

Hoffman, Paul. "Paul Hoffman on the Power of Music," *Gab with the Gurus with Connie Bennett* (February 4, 2011): http://www.blogtalkradio.com/gabwiththegurus/2011/02/04/paul-hoffman-on-the -power-of-music (accessed September 28, 2011).

Holthusen, Jordan et al. "ACE-Sponsored Research: Hooping—Effective Workout or Child's Play?" *American Council on Exercise* (January, 2011): http://www.acefitness.org/certifiednewsarticle/1094 /ace-sponsored-research-hooping-effective-workout (accessed September 28, 2011).

Home of the Glycemic Index. "What Is the Glycemic Index?": http://www.glycemicindex.com/ (accessed September 28, 2011).

Hsu, Wei-Chi and Hui-Ling Lai. "Effects of Music on Major Depression in Psychiatric Inpatients," *Archives of Psychiatric Nursing* (October 2004): http://www.psychiatricnursing.org/article /S0883-9417%2804%2900178-5/abstract (abstract accessed September 30, 2011).

Hwang, Kevin O. "Social Support in an Internet Weight Loss Community," *International Journal of Medical Informatics* 79, no. 1 (January 2010): 5–13. http://www.ncbi.nlm.nih.gov/pmc/articles /PMC3060773/?tool=pubmed (accessed October 16, 2011).

Hyman, Mark. "Sugar Addiction? It Might be Genetic," *Huffington Post* (February 6, 2011): http://www .huffingtonpost.com/dr-mark-hyman/sugar-addiction_b_819113.html (accessed September 28, 2011).

Hypoglycemia Support Foundation: www.hypoglcyemia.org (accessed October 7, 2011).

Jackson, Josh. "The 10 Best Sitcoms on TV Right Now," *Paste Magazine* (April 29, 2010): http://www .pastemagazine.com/blogs/lists/2010/04/the-10-best-sitcoms-on-tv-right-now.html (accessed September 28, 2011).

Jacob, Aglaee. "How Do I Consume Coconut Oil?" *Livestrong* (January 4, 2011): http://www.livestrong .com/article/349484-how-do-i-consume-coconut-oil/#ixzz1HFeDpl5p (accessed September 28, 2011).

Jain, Sarina. "Masala Bhangra Workout," *Masala Dance*: http://www.masaladance.com/EPK_2009.asp (accessed September 28, 2011).

Jameson, Marni. "A Reversal on Carbs," *Los Angeles Times* (December 20, 2010): http://articles.latimes .com/2010/dec/20/health/la-he-carbs-20101220 (accessed September 28, 2011).

Jegtvig, Shereen. "How Do I Convert Grams to Teaspoons?" *About.com* (October 8, 2011): http:// nutrition.about.com/od/askyournutritionist/f/gramconversion.htm (accessed October 16, 2011).

Jenkins, J. S. "The Mozart Effect," *Journal of the Royal Society of Medicine* 94, no. 4 (April 2001): 170– 172. http://www.ncbi.nlm.nih.gov/pmc/articles/PMC1281386/ (accessed September 28, 2011).

Jibrin, Janis. "More Zzzs for Better Blood Sugar," *The Dr. Oz Show*. Video. (June 28, 2010): http://www .doctoroz.com/videos/more-zzzs-better-blood-sugar (accessed September 28, 2011).

Johnson, C.S. et al. "Postprandial Thermogenesis is Increased 100% on a High-Protein Low-Fat Diet vs a High-Carbohydrate, Low-Fat diet in Healthy, Young Women," *Journal of the American College of Nutrition* 21, no. 1 (February 2002) : 55–61. http://www.jacn.org/content/21/1/55.long (accessed November 29, 2011).

Johnson, Gail. "Stressed? Help Is Just a Belly Breath Away," *Straight.com* (July 16, 2009): http://www .straight.com/article-240558/stressed-help-just-belly-breath-away (accessed September 28, 2011).

Johnson, Rachel et al. "Dietary Sugars Intake and Cardiovascular Health: A Scientific Statement from the American Heart Association," *Circulation* 120 (August 2009): 1011–1020. http://circ.ahajournals.org /content/120/11/1011.full.pdf+html (accessed October 16, 2011).

Johnson, Richard. "Dr. Mercola Interviews Dr. Richard Johnson on Fructose (Part 1 of 5)," *Mercola.com*. Video.: http://www.youtube.com/watch?v=ZjG5t4LN0jA (accessed November 21, 2011).

Johnson, Richard J. and Timothy Gower. *The Sugar Fix: The High-Fructose Fallout That Is Making You Fat and Sick*. New York: Pocket Books, 2009.

Johnston, Lauren. "Mini Review: Drinking Chia Fresca—The Runner's Super Beverage?" *New York Daily News* (September 8, 2010): http://www.nydailynews.com/blogs/running_dialogue/2010/09/mini -review-drinking-chia-fres.html (accessed September 28, 2011).

Jones, Martin. "The Mozart Effect," *Human Intelligence—Indiana University* (Fall 2003): http://www .indiana.edu/~intell/mozarteffect2.shtml#why (accessed September 28, 2011).

Josefson, Deborah. "High Insulin Levels Linked to Deaths from Breast Cancer," *British Medical Journal* 320, no. 7248 (June 3, 2000): 1496. http://www.ncbi.nlm.nih.gov/pmc/articles/PMC1118103/ (accessed October 1, 2011).

JustBeGood.net. "Free Downloads": http://www.justbegood.net/Downloads.htm (accessed September 28, 2011).

———. "Guided Metta Meditation": http://www.justbegood.net/Downloads/Other%20talks/Metta%20 Meditation.mp3 (accessed September 28, 2011).

———. "Index of /Downloads/Ajarn Brahm's Talks 3": http://www.justbegood.net/Downloads /Ajarn%20Brahm%27s%20Talks%203/ (accessed September 28, 2011).

Kabat-Zinn, Jon. *Coming to Our Senses: Healing Ourselves and the World Through Mindfulness.* United States: Hyperion, 2006.

———. "Jon Kabat-Zinn Speaking at CIHM Grand Opening Event," *Center for Investigating Healthy Minds*: http://www.investigatinghealthyminds.org/webcast/archive_jkz_event.html (accessed September 28, 2011).

———. *Wherever You Go, There You Are.* New York: Hyperion, 2005.

———. "Why Even Bother? The Importance of Meditation," *Spiritually Fit*: http://www.spirituallyfit.com /volume6/issue1/stories/jonkabatzinn.htm (accessed September 28, 2011).

Kaiser Permanente Center for Health Research. "CHR Study Finds Keeping Food Diaries Doubles Weight Loss": http://www.kpchr.org/research/public/news.aspx?newsid=3 (accessed September 28, 2011).

Kaizen Institute. "Masaaki Imai: Founder of the Kaizen Institute": http://www.kaizen.com/about-us /masaaki-imai-kaizen-pioneer-author-speaker.html (accessed September 28, 2011).

Kamen, Marina. "Marina Kamen: How Music Can Move You to Lose Weight, Etc," *Gab with the Gurus with Connie Bennett* (January 27, 2011): http://www.blogtalkradio.com/gabwiththegurus/2011/01/27 /marina-kamen-how-music-can-move-you-to-lose-weight-etc (accessed September 28, 2011).

———. E-mail follow-ups for "Marina Kamen's Sweet Success Story: How Music Helped Me Shed 100 Pounds."

Kant, Ashima et al. "Association of Breakfast Energy Density with Diet Quality and Body Mass Index in American Adults: National Health and Nutrition Examination Surveys, 1999–2004," *American Journal of Clinical Nutrition* 88, no. 5 (November 2008): 1396–1404. http://www.ajcn.org/content/88/5/1396 .long (abstract accessed September 28, 2011).

Katrandjian, Olivia. "Can't Beat the Fat and Sugar Cravings? Four Steps to Help You Kick Your Addictions," *ABC News* (February 3, 2011): http://abcnews.go.com/GMA/dr-mehmet-oz-beat-fat-sugar -addiction-detox/story?id=12823912 (accessed September 28, 2011).

Katsof, Rabbi Irwin. *How to Get Your Prayers Answered.* Hollywood, FL: Frederick Fell, 2002.

Kennedy, Dana. "Dana Kennedy: Creator of A Year Without Candy Blog," *Gab with the Gurus with Connie Bennett* (January 28, 2011): http://www.blogtalkradio.com/gabwiththegurus/2011/01/28/dana -kennedy-creator-of-a-year-without-candy-blog (accessed October 17, 2011).

———. E-mail correspondence for "Sweet Success Blogging Journey: A Year Without Candy."

Kessler, David A. *The End of Overeating: Taking Control of the Insatiable American Appetite.* New York: Rodale Books, 2010.

Kirsch, Irving. "Hypnotic Enhancement of Cognitive-Behavioral Weight Loss Treatments: Another Meta-Reanalysis," *Journal of Consulting and Clinical Psychology* 64, no. 33 (June 1996): 517–519. http:// psycnet.apa.org/journals/ccp/64/3/517/ (abstract accessed September 28, 2011).

Kivinen, Michael. "Hypnosis: It's Not Just a Stage Act," Presentation as part of the 2009–2010 Psychology Lecture Series. Video. (March 8, 2010): http://www.youtube.com/watch?v=MKRnPn7khtU (accessed September 28, 2011).

Kolata, Gina. "Lactic Acid Is Not Muscles' Foe, It's Fuel," *The New York Times* (May 16, 2006): http://www.nytimes.com/2006/05/16/health/nutrition/16run.html (accessed September 28, 2011).

Korn, Danna. "Do You Have Gluten Problems," *Gab with the Gurus with Connie Bennett* (January 20, 2011): http://www.blogtalkradio.com/gabwiththegurus/2011/01/20/do-you-have-gluten-problems-with-danna-korn (accessed October 16, 2011).

Kovacs, Jenny Stamos. "Lose Weight While You Sleep!" *Glamour* (February 2, 2009): http://www.glamour.com/magazine/2009/02/lose-weight-while-you-sleep?currentPage=1 (accessed September 28, 2011).

———. "Snooze and Lose! Sleep Off Those Extra Pounds," *The Today Show* (February 9, 2009): http://today.msnbc.msn.com/id/29057007/ns/today-today_health/ (accessed September 28, 2011).

Kumanyika, Shiriki et al. "Trial of Family and Friend Support for Weight Loss in African American Adults," *Archives of Internal Medicine* 169, no. 19 (October 26, 2009): 1795–1804. http://archinte.ama-assn.org/cgi/content/abstract/169/19/1795 (accessed October 17, 2011).

Laddau, Meryl Davids. "Do You Need a Health Coach? Pointers from the Pros," *Health Coach Training* (February 18, 2011): http://www.healthcoachtraining.com/news/news2011_02_18.shtml (accessed September 28, 2011).

LaForgia, J. et al. "Effects of Exercise Intensity and Duration on the Excess Post-Exercise Oxygen Consumption," *Journal of Sports Science* 24, no. 12 (December 2006): 1247–1264. http://www.bodyrecomposition.com/research-review/research-review-effects-of-exercise-intensity-and-duration-on-the-excess-post-exercise-oxygen-consumption.html (accessed September 28, 2011).

Lairon, Denis. "Nutritional Quality and Safety of Organic Food: A Review," *Agronomy for Sustainable Development* 30, no. 1 (March 2010): 33–41. http://www.agronomy-journal.org/index.php?option=com_article&access=doi&doi=10.1051/agro/2009019&Itemid=129 (accessed September 28, 2011).

LaRosa, John. "U.S. Sleep Aids Market Grows To $23 Billion, As Americans Battle Insomnia, Sleep Disorders," *PRWeb* (June 9, 2008): http://www.prweb.com/releases/2008/06/prweb1006354.htm (accessed September 28, 2011).

Larsson, S.C. "Processed Meat Consumption, Dietary Nitrosamines and Stomach Cancer Risk in a Cohort of Swedish Women," *International Journal of Cancer* 119, no. 4 (August 15, 2006): 915–919.

Laursen, P.B. "Training for Intense Exercise Performance: High-Intensity or High-Volume Training?" *Scandinavian Journal of Medicine & Science in Sports* 20 (October 2010): 1–10. Abstract Only: http://www.ncbi.nlm.nih.gov/pubmed/20840557 (accessed September 30, 2011).

Layton, Julia. "Is It True That if You Do Anything for Three Weeks It Will Become a Habit?" *Discovery Fit & Health:* http://health.howstuffworks.com/mental-health/human-nature/behavior/form-a-habit.htm (accessed September 28, 2011).

Ledwell, Natalie. "How to Make a Mind Movie," *Sweeter Holiday Summit with Connie Bennett* Episode #38 (December 15, 2010): http://instantteleseminar.com/?eventid=16530096 (accessed September 30, 2011).

Lee, Rebecca. "The Mozart Effect," *ABC News* (May 25, 2007): http://abcnews.go.com/Technology/story?id=3213324&page=2 (accessed September 28, 2011).

Lien, Lars et al. "Consumption of Soft Drinks and Hyperactivity, Mental Distress, and Conduct Problems Among Adolescents in Oslo, Norway," *American Journal of Public Health* 10 (2006): 1815-1820. http://ajph.aphapublications.org/cgi/content/full/96/10/1815?view=long&pmid=17008578 (accessed November 20, 2011).

Look, Carol. "Emotional Freedom Techniques," *Attracting Abundance* (2010): http://cdn.attracting abundance.com/eft/wp-content/uploads/EFT-Directions.pdf (accessed September 28, 2011).

———. "How to Attract Abundance this Holiday Season and Beyond," *Sweeter Holiday Summit with Connie Bennett* Segment #31 (December 14, 2010): http://InstantTeleseminar.com/?eventid=16293153

———. "What is EFT?" *Attracting Abundance*: http://www.attractingabundance.com/eft/what-is-eft/ (accessed September 28, 2011).

Loux, Renee. "Top 10 Reasons to Go Organic," *Prevention* (September 27, 2006): http://www .prevention.com/health/nutrition/healthy-eating-tips/organic-foods-health-and-diet/article/2426d08f88 803110VgnVCM20000012281eac_(accessed October 16, 2011).

Ludwig, David et al. "Relation between consumption of sugar-sweetened drinks and childhood obesity: a prospective, observational analysis," *The Lancet* 357 (February 17, 2001): 505–508. http://nepc .colorado.edu/files/lancet.pdf (accessed September 28, 2011).

Luskin, Fred. "Learn to Forgive with Dr. Fred Luskin," *Gab with the Gurus with Connie Bennett* (August 3, 2011): http://www.blogtalkradio.com/gabwiththegurus/2010/08/03/learn-to-forgive-with-dr-fred-luskin (accessed October 16, 2011).

Lustig, Robert. "Childhood Obesity: Behavioral Aberration or Biochemical Drive? Reinterpreting the First Law of Thermodynamics," *Nature Clinical Practice Endocrinology and Metabolism* 22, no. 8 (August 2006): 447–458. http://www.ncbi.nlm.nih.gov/pubmed/16932334 (accessed September 28, 2011).

———. "The Fructose Epidemic," Video. (January 26, 2010): http://www.youtube.com /watch?v=277MKP7uV5g (accessed September 28, 2011).

———. "Sugar: The Bitter Truth," Video. (July 30, 2009): http://www.youtube.com/watch?v =dBnniua6-oM (accessed September 28, 2011).

———. "Sweet Addiction," Video. (May 17, 2010): http://www.youtube.com/watch?v=yHoIDMOB-_A (accessed September 28, 2011).

———. "The Trouble with Fructose": http://www.slideshare.net/ancestralhealth/ahs-slidesrobert-lustig (accessed September 28, 2011).

M., Michele. Phone interview and e-mail follow-ups for "Michele M.'s Sweet Success Story: How I Quit Sugar & Rediscovered My Marriage."

Ma, Y. et al. "Association Between Eating Patterns and Obesity in a Free-living US Adult Population," *American Journal of Epidemiology* 158, no. 1 (July 1, 2003): 85–92. http://www.ncbi.nlm.nih.gov /pubmed/12835290 (abstract accessed September 28, 2011).

Maas, James B. "Learn About the Power of Sleep and Gratitude," *Gab with the Gurus with Connie Bennett* (September 21, 2010): http://www.blogtalkradio.com/gabwiththegurus/2010/09/21/learn-about-the -power-of-sleep-gratitude-1 (accessed September 28, 2011).

# Bibliography

Macatee, Rebecca. "Kevin Smith Lost 65 Pounds After Being Kicked Off Airplane for Being Too Fat," *PopEater* (February 8, 2011): http://www.popeater.com/2011/02/08/kevin-smith-weight-loss/ (accessed September 28, 2011).

Magee, Elaine. "Good Carbs, Bad Carbs: Why Carbohydrates Matter to You," *WebMD* (October 30, 2008): http://www.webmd.com/food-recipes/features/carbohydrates (accessed September 28, 2011).

Malik, V.S. "Sugar-Sweetened Beverages and Risk of Metabolic Syndrome and Type 2 Diabetes: A Meta-analysis," *Diabetes Care* 33, no. 11 (November 2010): 2477–2483. http://www.ncbi.nlm.nih.gov/pubmed/20693348 (accessed abstract October 1, 2011).

Maltz, Maxwell. *Psycho-Cybernetics: A New Way to Get More Living Out of Life*. New York: Pocket Books, 1989. Originally published in 1960 by Simon & Schuster.

Maraney, Saul. "Interview with Dr. Hew Len," WhatIsHo'oponopono.com: http://whatishooponopono.com/Interview_with_Dr_Hew_Len.htm (accessed September 28, 2011).

Maratos, Anna et al. "Music Therapy for Depression," *The Cochrane Library* (January 21, 2009): http://onlinelibrary.wiley.com/o/cochrane/clsysrev/articles/CD004517/frame.html (abstract accessed September 28, 2011).

Mars, Brigitte. "Herbs to Spice Up Your Holiday Season," *Sweeter Holiday Summit with Connie Bennett* Segment #26 (December 9, 2010): http://InstantTeleseminar.com/?eventid=16292901 (accessed September 30, 2011).

Martinez, Richard. E-mail follow-ups for "Richard Martinez's Zumba Sweet Success Story: 75 Pounds Fell Off & My Confidence Soared."

Mastroianni, Thomas. "The Mozart Effect—Duality in Human Cognitive Processing": www.thomasmastroianni.com/docs/MozartEffectduality.doc (accessed September 30, 2011).

Mayo Clinic, The. "Cardiovascular Surgery Healing Enhancement Program": http://www.mayoclinic.org/cv-surgery-healing-enhancement/types.html (accessed September 28, 2011).

———. "Yoga: Tap Into the Many Health Benefits": http://www.mayoclinic.com/health/yoga/CM00004 (accessed September 28, 2011).

McGhee, Paul. "Humor and Laughter Strengthen Your Immune System." *The Laughter Remedy* (January 25, 2011): http://www.laughterremedy.com/2011/01/humor-and-laughter-strengthen-your-immune-system/ (accessed September 28, 2011).

McIver, Shane et al. "'Overeating Is Not About the Food': Women Describe Their Experience of a Yoga Treatment Program for Binge Eating." *Qualitative Health Research* 104, no. 9 (September 2009): 1234–1245, http://qhr.sagepub.com/content/19/9/1234 (abstract accessed September 28, 2011).

Meatless Mondays. "Nutritional FAQ": http://www.meatlessmonday.com/nutritional-faq/ (accessed November 20, 2011).

MedlinePlus Medical Dictionary. "Triglyceride Level": http://www.nlm.nih.gov/medlineplus/ency/article/003493.htm (accessed October 15, 2011).

Mercola, Joseph. "Americans Don't Drink Enough Water," *Mercola* (June 10, 2000): http://articles.mercola.com/sites/articles/archive/2000/06/10/water-part-one.aspx (accessed September 28, 2011).

———. "Basic Steps to Your Emotional Freedom," *Mercola*: http://eft.mercola.com/ (accessed September 28, 2011).

———. "Want to Burn More Fat during Exercise? Take a Break," *Mercola*. Video. (July 20, 2007): http://articles.mercola.com/sites/articles/archive/2007/07/20/want-to-burn-more-fat-during-exercise-take-a-break.aspx?PageIndex=2 (accessed September 28, 2011).

Merendino Jr., John. "Sugar Highs Explained," *The Dr. Oz Show*. Video. (June 28, 2010): http://www.doctoroz.com/videos/sugar-highs-explained (accessed September 28, 2011).

Migliore, Marilyn Ann. *The Hunger Within: An Enlightening Journey to Recovery from Compulsive Eating*. New York. Revised and reprinted by arrangement with Random House, 2008.

Miller, M. and W.F. Fry. "The Effect of Mirthful Laughter on the Human Cardiovascular System," *Medical Hypotheses* 73, no. 5 (November 2009): 636–639. http://www.ncbi.nlm.nih.gov/pubmed/19477604 (abstract accessed September 28, 2011).

Miller, A. and K. Adeli "Dietary Fructose and the Metabolic Syndrome," *Current Opinion in Gastroenterology* 24, no. 2 (March 2008): 204–209. http://www.ncbi.nlm.nih.gov/pubmed/18301272 (abstract accessed October 14, 2011).

Mindfulness Solution, The. "Meditation Downloads": http://www.mindfulness-solution.com/DownloadMeditations.html (accessed September 30, 2011).

Monique, Tiffany. "Tiffany Monique—Beyoncé Back-Up Singer Shares Weight Loss Story," *Gab with the Gurus with Connie Bennett* (March 2, 2011): http://www.blogtalkradio.com/gabwiththegurus/2011/03/02/tiffany-monique---beyonce-back-up-singer-shares-weight-loss-story (accessed September 28, 2011).

———. E-mails for "Monique's Sweet Success Story: The Backup Singer for Beyoncé Sheds Weight with Support at SparkPeople."

Monteleone, P. et al. "Circadian Rhythms and Treatment Implications in Depression," *Progress in Neuro-Psychopharmacology & Biological Psychiatry* 35, no. 7 (August 5, 2010):1569–1574. http://www.ncbi.nlm.nih.gov/pubmed/20691746 (abstract accessed September 28, 2011).

Moore, Jimmy. "Eat Your Way to Health & Weight Loss with Jimmy Moore & Dr. Ronald Hoffman," *Gab with the Gurus with Connie Bennett* (Feb. 24, 2010): http://www.blogtalkradio.com/gabwiththegurus/2010/02/24/eat-your-way-to-health-weight-loss. (accessed October 6, 2011).

———. E-mails for "Jimmy Moore's Sweet Success Story: My Wife's Loving Support Helped Me Lose 180 Pounds."

———. "Jimmy's Interview with Dr. Robert Lustig from 'Sugar: The Bitter Truth.'" *Jimmy Moore's Livin' La Vida Lo-Carb* (July 5, 2010): http://www.livinlowcarbdiscussion.com/showthread.php?tid=4855 (accessed September 28, 2011).

Morain, Claudia. "Emmons: Studying New Science of Gratitude," *UC Davis* (November 2, 2007): http://dateline.ucdavis.edu/dl_detail.lasso?id=9839 (accessed September 28, 2011).

Morrison, Jeffrey A. *Cleanse Your Body, Clear Your Mind: Eliminate Environmental Toxins to Lose Weight, Increase Energy, and Reverse Illness in 30 Days or Less*. New York: Hudson Street Press, 2011.

# Bibliography

Mueller, Jen. "Confession: My Sugar Addiction has Returned," SparkPeople.com (December 17, 2010): http://www.dailyspark.com/blog.asp?post=confession_my_sugar_addiction_has_returned (accessed October 7, 2011).

Mueller, Noel et al. "Soft Drink and Juice Consumption and Risk of Pancreatic Cancer: The Singapore Chinese Health Study," *Cancer Epidemiology Biomarkers & Prevention* 19 (February 1, 2010): 447–455. http://cebp.aacrjournals.org/content/19/2/447.full (accessed October 16, 2011).

Muti, Paola et al. "Fasting Glucose Is a Risk Factor for Breast Cancer: A Prospective Study," *Cancer Epidemiology Biomarkers & Prevention* 11 (November 2002): 1361–1368. http://cebp.aacrjournals.org /content/11/11/1361.abstract (accessed October 16, 2011).

Nagle, C.M. et al. "Carbohydrate Intake, Glycemic Load, Glycemic Index, and Risk of Ovarian Cancer," *Annals of Oncology* 22, no. 6 (2011): 1332–1338 first published online December 3, 2010. http:// annonc.oxfordjournals.org/content/22/6/1332.abstract (accessed October 1, 2011).

Nakamura, P.M. et al. "Effects of Preferred and Nonpreferred Music on Continuous Cycling Exercise Performance," *Perceptual and Motor Skills* 110, no. 1 (February 11, 2010): 257–264. http://www.ncbi.nlm .nih.gov/pubmed/20391890 (abstract accessed September 28, 2011).

National Association of Anorexia Nervosa and Associated Disorders, Inc. "Eating Disorder Statistics": http://www.anad.org/get-information/about-eating-disorders/eating-disorders-statistics/ (accessed September 28, 2011).

National Cancer Institute. "Acrylamide in Food and Cancer Risk": http://www.cancer.gov/cancertopics /factsheet/Risk/acrylamide-in-food (accessed October 15, 2011).

National Confectioners Association. "New Study Shows You Can Have Your Candy and Eat it Too—Without Adverse Health Effects" (March 29, 2011): http://www.candyusa.com/IndustryResources/PRdetail .cfm?ItemNumber=3909 (accessed September 28, 2011).

———. "New Study Finds Candy Consumption Not Associated with Negative Health Outcomes," (April 20, 2009): http://www.candyusa.com/IndustryResources/PRdetail.cfm?ItemNumber=1239 (accessed September 28, 2011).

National Institute of Neurological Disorders and Stroke. "Brain Basics: Understanding Sleep" (May 21, 2007): http://www.ninds.nih.gov/disorders/brain_basics/understanding_sleep.htm (accessed September 28, 2011).

National Weight Control Registry, The. "NWCR Facts": http://www.nwcr.ws/Research/default.htm (accessed September 28, 2011).

Naturally Simple Living. "Celebrations, Moderation, and the Standard American Diet," (July 28, 2011): http://naturallysimple.org/living/2011/07/18/celebrations-moderation-and-the-standard-american-diet/ (accessed September 28, 2011).

Neff, Kristin. "Guided Self Compassion Meditations," Self-Compassion.org: http://www.self-compassion .org/guided-self-compassion-meditations-mp3.html (accessed September 30, 2011).

———. "Loving-Kindness Meditation," Self-Compassion.org: http://www.self-compassion.org/LKM .MP3 (accessed September 23, 2011).

———. *Self-Compassion: Stop Beating Yourself Up and Leave Insecurity Behind.* New York: HarperCollins, 2011.

———. "Why Compassion Trumps Self-Esteem," *Greater Good: The Science of a Meaningful Life* (May 27, 2011): http://greatergood.berkeley.edu/article/item/try_selfcompassion/ (accessed September 28, 2011).

Neff, Kristin and Christopher Germer. "Integrating Mindfulness and Self-Compassion," *Center for Mindfulness in Medicine, Health Care, and Society* (April 7, 2010): http://www.mindfulnet.org/NeffGermer_Self-CompassnHandout_Apr10.pdf (accessed October 1, 2011).

Neporent, Liz. "Lack of Sleep Linked to Childhood Obesity," *ABC News* (January 24, 2011): http://abcnews.go.com/Health/lack-weekend-catch-sleep-risk-childhood-obesity/story?id=12743677 (accessed September 28, 2011).

Nerurkar, Aditi. "Meditation vs. Medication: Which Should You Choose?" *Huffington Post* (February 11, 2011): http://www.huffingtonpost.com/aditi-nerurkar-md-mph/benefits-of-meditation-_b_820177.html (accessed September 28, 2011).

Nettleson, J.A. et al. "Diet Soda Intake and Risk of Incident Metabolic Syndrome and Type 2 Diabetes in the Multi-Ethnic Study of Atherosclerosis (MESA)," *Diabetes Care* 32, no. 4 (April 2009): 688–694. http://www.ncbi.nlm.nih.gov/pubmed/19151203 (abstract accessed September 28, 2011).

Newby-Clark, Ian. "Creatures of Habit: Effective Advice for Lasting Habit Change. What Went Right? You Focused on One Habit!?" *Psychology Today* (June 25, 2010): http://www.psychologytoday.com/blog/creatures-habit/201006/what-went-right-you-focused-one-habit (accessed September 30, 2011).

———. "Five Things You Need to Know About Effective Habit Change," *ZenHabits* (November 5, 2007): http://zenhabits.net/five-things-you-need-to-know-about-effective-habit-change/ (accessed September 28, 2011).

———. "Plans and Predictions for Exercise Frequency Change," *Basic and Applied Social Psychology* 27, no. 2 (2005): 97–106. http://www.tandfonline.com/doi/abs/10.1207/s15324834basp2702_1#preview (abstract accessed September 28, 2011).

Nhat Hanh, Thich. *The Miracle of Mindfulness: An Introduction to the Practice of Meditation.* Boston: Beacon Press, 1999.

Nichols, Nicole. "Study: Your Method of Food Tracking Can Help or Hurt Your Weight Loss," *DailySpark* (March 9, 2011): http://www.dailyspark.com/blog.asp?post=study_your_choice_of_food_diary_can_help_or_hurt_your_weight_loss (accessed September 28, 2011).

Nielsen, Samara Joy et al. "Trends in Energy Intake in U.S. Between 1977 and 1996: Similar Shifts Seen Across Age Groups," *Obesity Research* 10, no. 5 (May 2002): 370–378. http://www.cpc.unc.edu/projects/nutrans/publications/SamaraAllages-trends-OR.pdf (accessed September 28, 2011).

Norris, Jeffrey. "Sugar is a Poison, Says UCSF Obesity Expert," *UCSF* (June 25, 2009): http://www.ucsf.edu/news/2009/06/8187/obesity-and-metabolic-syndrome-driven-fructose-sugar-diet (accessed September 28, 2011).

Nourishing Days. "Phytic Acid: Defining and Dealing With a Common Antinutrient" (September 14, 2010): http://www.nourishingdays.com/2010/09/what-is-phytic-acid/ (accessed September 28, 2011).

# Bibliography

The NPD Group. "31 Million U.S. Consumers Skip Breakfast Each Day Reports NPD," NPDGroup.com (October 11, 2011): http://www.npdgroup.com/wps/portal/npd/us/news/pressreleases /pr_111011b/!ut/p/c5/04_SB8K8xL (accessed November 23, 2011).

Nybo, L. et al. "High-Intensity Training Versus Traditional Exercise Interventions for Promoting Health," *Medicine & Science in Sports & Exercise* 42, no. 10 (October 2010): 1951–1958. http://www.ncbi.nlm .nih.gov/pubmed/20195181 (accessed September 30, 2011).

Oexman, Robert. "Sleep Deprived? Depressed? There's a Connection," *Gab with the Gurus with Connie Bennett* (December 22, 2010): http://www.blogtalkradio.com/gabwiththegurus/2010/12/22 /sleep-deprived-depressed-theres-a-connection (accessed October 16, 2011).

Ogden, Cynthia L., and Margaret Carroll. "Prevalence of Obesity Among Children and Adolescents: United States, Trends 1963–1965 Through 2007–2008," *Centers for Disease Control* (June 2010): http:// www.cdc.gov/nchs/data/hestat/obesity_child_07_08/obesity_child_07_08.pdf (accessed September 28, 2011).

———. "Prevalence of Overweight, Obesity, and Extreme Obesity Among Adults: United States, Trends 1960–1962 Through 2007–2008," *Centers for Disease Control* (June 2010): http://www.cdc.gov/NCHS /data/hestat/obesity_adult_07_08/obesity_adult_07_08.pdf (accessed September 28, 2011).

O'Keefe, James et al. "Exercise Like a Hunter-Gatherer: A Prescription for Organic Physical Fitness," *Progress in Cardiovascular Diseases* 53 (2011): 471–479. http://thepaleodiet.com/wp-content /uploads/2011/02/OKeefe-Cordain-2011.pdf (accessed October 16, 2011).

O'Leary, Noreen. "Soft-Drink Consumption Continues to Decline," *Adweek* (March 30, 2010): http:// www.brandweek.com/bw/content_display/news-and-features/packaged-goods/e3iedc670800607 df6c191cf7d4164ab322 (accessed September 28, 2011).

Ortiz, Edward. "New Study Says Mozart's Music Has Little Effect on Brain Performance," *The Sacramento Bee* (May 13, 2010): http://blogs.sacbee.com/mt/mt-search.cgi?blog_id=11&tag=Frances%20H.%20 Rauscher&limit=20&IncludeBlogs=11 (accessed September 28, 2011).

Ortner, Jessica. "Tapping World Summit," Video. http://www.youtube.com/watch?v=0sLaPUppAxo (accessed October 16, 2011).

Ortner, Nick et al. *The Tapping Solution: The Revolution Starts Within.* DVD (July 1, 2009), Try It Productions.

Overeaters Anonymous: http://www.oa.org/ (accessed September 28, 2011).

Oz, Mehmet. "Health Coach Kudos from Dr. Oz," *Larry King Live.* Video. http://www.youtube.com /watch?v=ufyucZpdyRY (accessed September 28, 2011).

———. "How You Can Stay Young and Youthful," appearance on *Stop Sugar Shock Radio* (precursor to *Gab with the Gurus with Connie Bennett*) (October 30, 2007): http://www.blogtalkradio.com/stop sugarshock/2007/10/30/how-to-stay-young-with-dr-mehmet-oz (accessed October 7, 2011).

———. "Sugar Shock," Oprah Radio (March 21, 2007): http://www.oprah.com/health/Sugar-Shock (accessed October 7, 2011).

Paleo Diet, The. "About the Paleo Diet," *Thepaleodiet.com:* http://thepaleodiet.com/about/ (accessed September 28, 2011).

Paltrow, Gwyneth. "Overcoming Sugar Addiction," *GOOP*, http://goop.com/newsletter/103/en/ (accessed September 28, 2011).

Parker-Pope, Tara. "Go Easy on Yourself, a New Wave of Research Urges," *The New York Times* (February 28, 2011): http://well.blogs.nytimes.com/2011/02/28/go-easy-on-yourself-a-new-wave-of-research-urges/ (accessed September 30, 2011).

————. "Late Night Eating Linked to Weight Gain," *The New York Times* (September 3, 2009): http://well.blogs.nytimes.com/2009/09/03/late-night-eating-linked-to-weight-gain/ (accessed September 28, 2011).

————. "Six Meaningless Claims on Food Labels," *The New York Times* (January 28, 2010): http://well.blogs.nytimes.com/2010/01/28/six-meaningless-claims-on-food-labels/ (accessed September 28, 2011).

————. "Using Music to Lift Depression's Veil," *The New York Times* (January 24, 2008): http://well.blogs.nytimes.com/2008/01/24/using-music-to-lift-depressions-veil/ (accessed September 28, 2011).

Patel, Sanjay R. "Sleep—An Affair of the Heart," *Sleep* 32, no. 3 (March 1, 2009): 289–290. http://www.ncbi.nlm.nih.gov/pmc/articles/PMC2647781/ (accessed September 28, 2011).

Peck, Peggy. "ASH: Daily Doses of Bach and Breathing Lower Blood Pressure," *MedPage Today* (May 23, 2008): http://www.medpagetoday.com/MeetingCoverage/ASH/9597 (accessed September 28, 2011).

Peel, Elizabeth et al. "Type 2 Diabetes and Dog Walking: Patients' Longitudinal Perspectives About Implementing and Sustaining Physical Activity," *British Journal of General Practice* 60, no. 577 (August 2010): 570–577. http://www.ncbi.nlm.nih.gov/pmc/articles/PMC2913737/ (accessed September 28, 2011).

PepsiCo Inc. "Caffeine," *Pepsibeveragefacts.com.* Updated September 15, 2011: http://www.pepsicobeveragefacts.com/caffeine.php (accessed September 28, 2011).

Philpott, Tom. "3 Ways Scientific American Got the Organic Ag Story Wrong," *Mother Jones* (July 25, 2011): http://motherjones.com/tom-philpott/2011/07/organic-agriculture (accessed September 28, 2011).

Phinney, Stephen et al. "Carbohydrate Restriction Has a More Favorable Impact on the Metabolic Syndrome than a Low Fat Diet," *Lipids* 44, no. 4 (April 2009): 297–309. http://www.springerlink.com/content/v57212m331741w24/ (accessed October 16, 2011).

Physicians Committee for Responsible Medicine. "New Spoof of Milk Mustache Ad Spotlights Lactose Intolerance." http://www.pcrm.org/search/?cid=1944 (accessed Nov. 27, 2011).

Pick, Marcelle. "Caffeine and Your Adrenals—Could They Be Paying Dearly?" *Women to Women* (April 15, 2011): http://www.womentowomen.com/adrenalhealth/caffeine-stress-adrenalfatigue.aspx (accessed September 28, 2011).

————. "Caffeine Pros and Cons: Effects of Caffeine on Your Body," *Women to Women* (April 20, 2011): http://www.womentowomen.com/fatigueandstress/effectsofcaffeine.aspx (accessed September 28, 2011).

————. "Deep Breathing—The Truly Essential Exercise," *Women to Women* (April 20, 2011): http://www.womentowomen.com/fatigueandstress/deepbreathing.aspx (accessed September 28, 2011).

# Bibliography

Pizer, Ann. "Yoga Style Guide," *About.com* (August 21, 2011): http://yoga.about.com/od /typesofyoga/a/yogatypes.htm (accessed September 28, 2011).

Plante, Thomas G. et al. "Exercising with an iPod, Friend, or Neither: Which is Better for Psychological Benefits?" *American Journal of Health Behavior* 35, no. 2 (2011): 199–208. http://www.ajhb.org/issues/2 011/2/02MarApr0711Plante.pdf (abstract accessed September 28, 2011).

Pollack, Andrew. "Fuel Lines of Tumors are New Target," *The New York Times* (November 29, 2010): http://www.nytimes.com/2010/11/30/health/30cancer.html (accessed September 28, 2011).

Pollan, Michael. *Food Rules: An Eater's Manual.* New York: Penguin, 2009.

Pou, Jackie. "The Dirty Dozen and Clean 15 of Produce," *PBS* (May 13, 2010): http://www.pbs.org/wnet /need-to-know/health/the-dirty-dozen-and-clean-15-of-produce/616/ (accessed September 28, 2011).

PubMed Health. "Hardening of the Arteries": http://www.ncbi.nlm.nih.gov/pubmedhealth /PMH0001224/ (accessed October 15, 2011).

Pusztai, Arpad. "Genetically Modified Foods: Are They a Risk to Human/Animal Health?" *ActionBioscience.org* (a resource of the American Institute of Biological Sciences): http://www.actionbioscience.org /biotech/pusztai.html (accessed September 30, 2011).

Quan, Stuart F. et al. "Healthy Sleep Education: A Salve for Obesity?" *Journal of Clinical Sleep Medicine* 6, no. 1 (February 15, 2010); 18–19. http://www.ncbi.nlm.nih.gov/pmc/articles/PMC2823271/ (accessed September 28, 2011).

Rae-Dupree, Janet. "Can You Become a Creature of New Habits?" *The New York Times* (May 4, 2008) http://www.nytimes.com/2008/05/04/business/04unbox.html (accessed September 28, 2011).

Reinagel, Monica. "What are the Benefits of Coconut Oil?" *Nutrition Diva* (July 22, 2009): http:// nutritiondiva.quickanddirtytips.com/benefits-of-coconut-oil.aspx (accessed September 28, 2011).

Reynolds, Gretchen. "What's the Single Best Exercise?" *The New York Times* (April 15, 2011): http:// www.nytimes.com/2011/04/17/magazine/mag-17exercise-t.html (accessed September 28, 2011).

Richardson, Caroline R. et al. "An Online Community Improves Adherence in an Internet-Mediated Walking Program. Part 1: Results of a Randomized Controlled Trial," *Journal of Medical Internet Research* 12, no. 4 (December 17, 2010): http://www.ncbi.nlm.nih.gov/pmc/articles/PMC3056526/ (accessed September 28, 2011).

Richardson, Cheryl. *The Art of Extreme Self-Care: Transform Your Life One Month at a Time.* Carlsbad, CA: Hay House, 2009.

———. *Take Time for Your Life: A Personal Coach's 7-Step Program for Creating the Life You Want.* New York: Three Rivers Press, 1999.

Romine, Stepfanie. "Meet Tiffany, a SparkPeople Success Story and the Next Big Star!" *Daily Spark* (February 10, 2011): http://www.dailyspark.com/blog.asp?post=meet_tiffany_a_sparkpeople_success_story _and_the_next_big_star (accessed September 28, 2011).

Rourke, David. "Lose Weight and Conquer Addictions Using EFT With David Rourke," *Gab with the Gurus with Connie Bennett* (December 30, 2010): http://www.blogtalkradio.com/gabwiththe gurus/2010/12/30/lose-weight-conquer-addictions-using-eft-with-davi (accessed September 28, 2011).

Sacks, Frank M. et al. "Comparison of Weight-Loss Diets with Different Compositions of Fat, Protein, and Carbohydrates," *The New England Journal of Medicine* 360 (February 26, 2009): 859–873. http://www.nejm.org/doi/full/10.1056/NEJMoa0804748 (accessed September 28, 2011).

Salmerón, Jorge et al. "Dietary Fiber, Glycemic Load, and Risk of Non-insulin-dependent Diabetes Mellitus in Women," *Journal of the American Medical Association* 277, no. 6 (February 12, 1997): 472–477. http://prh.com.mx/biblioteca/diabetes/18.%20Dietary%20Fiber,%20Glycemic%20Load,%20and%20 risk%20of%20non%20insulin%20dependent%20diabetes%20mellitus%20in%20women.pdf (accessed September 28, 2011).

Salzberg, Sharon. "Facets of Metta," *Vipassana.com* (1995): http://www.vipassana.com/meditation /facets_of_metta.php (accessed September 28, 2011).

———. "Glossary," SharonSalzberg.com: http://www.sharonsalzberg.com/glossary (accessed September 28, 2011).

———. "Meditations," SharonSalzberg.com: http://www.sharonsalzberg.com/meditations (accessed September 28, 2011).

———. "Opening the Heart: Use the Metta, or Lovingkindness, Meditation to Cultivate a Deep Sense of Caring for Self and for All of Creation," *Beliefnet*: http://www.beliefnet.com/Health/2000/07/Opening -The-Heart.aspx (accessed September 28, 2011).

———. "Sharon Salzberg's Dharma Talks," *DharmaSeed.org:* http://www.dharmaseed.org/teacher/165 (accessed September 28, 2011).

Sample, Ian. "Organic Food is Healthier: Study," *The Guardian* (October 28, 2007): http://www .guardian.co.uk/science/2007/oct/29/organics.sciencenews (accessed October 16, 2011).

Schaler, Jeffrey A. *Addiction Is a Choice.* Chicago: Open Court, 2000.

Schernhammer, Eva S. et al. "Sugar-Sweetened Soft Drink Consumption and Risk of Pancreatic Cancer in Two Prospective Cohorts," *Cancer, Epidemiology, Biomarkers & Prevention* 14 (September 2005): 2098. http://cebp.aacrjournals.org/content/14/9/2098.full (accessed October 1, 2011).

Schulze, M.B. et al. "Sugar-Sweetened Beverages, Weight Gain, and Incidence of Type 2 Diabetes in Young and Middle-Aged Women," *Journal of the American Medical Association* 292, no. 8 (August 25, 2004): 927–934. http://www.ncbi.nlm.nih.gov/pubmed/15328324 (accessed October 1, 2011).

Schwarz, Joyce. "Build a Vision Now for Next Year's Success," *Sweeter Holiday Summit with Connie Bennett* Session #33. Private Program (December14, 2010): http://InstantTeleseminar .com/?eventid=16293342 (accessed September 30, 2011).

Science Daily. "High Sugar Consumption May Increase Risk Factors for Heart Disease in American Teenagers": http://www.sciencedaily.com/releases/2011/01/110110164929.htm (accessed September 30, 2011).

———. "Keeping a Food Diary Doubles Diet Weight Loss, Study Suggests": http://www.sciencedaily .com/releases/2008/07/080708080738.htm (accessed September 28, 2011).

———. "Mozart's Music Does Not Make You Smarter, Study Finds" (May 10, 2010): http://www .sciencedaily.com/releases/2010/05/100510075415.htm (accessed September 28, 2011).

————. "Mozart Therapy: A Sonata a Day Keeps the Doctor Away" (January 8, 2010): http://www .sciencedaily.com/releases/2010/01/100107132551.htm (accessed September 28, 2011).

Seiler, Bill and Ellen Beth Levitt. "Joyful Music May Promote Heart Health, According to University of Maryland School of Medicine Study," *University of Maryland Medical Center* (November 11, 2008): http://www.umm.edu/news/releases/music-cardiovascular.htm (accessed September 28, 2011).

Seliger, Susan. "'Superfoods' Everyone Needs," *WebMD:* http://www.webmd.com/diet/features/super foods-everyone-needs (accessed September 28, 2011).

Sengupta, Somini. "Extreme Mumbai, Without Bollywood's Filtered Lens," *The New York Times* (November 11, 2008): http://www.nytimes.com/2008/11/16/movies/16seng.html (accessed September 28, 2011).

Share Guide: The Holistic Health Magazine and Health Directory. "Interview with Ann Louise Gittleman": http://www.shareguide.com/Gittleman.html (accessed September 28, 2011).

Shimoff, Marci and Carol Kline. *Happy for No Reason: 7 Steps to Being Happy from the inside Out.* New York: Free Press, 2008.

Siegel, Bernie S. *365 Prescriptions for the Soul: Daily Messages of Inspiration, Hope, and Love.* Novato, CA: New World Library, 2009.

————. "Bernie Siegel on Miracles." *Gab with the Gurus with Connie Bennett.* (October 19, 2011): http:// www.blogtalkradio.com/gabwiththegurus/2011/10/19/bernie-siegel-on-miracles (accessed November 29, 2011).

Siegel, Ronald. "The Mindfulness Solution to Holiday Stress," *Sweeter Holiday Summit with Connie Bennett* Segment #15 of private teleseminar series (Nov. 30, 2010): http://InstantTeleseminar .com/?eventid=16230216. (accessed September 30, 2011).

Silverglade, Bruce and Ilene Ringel Heller. "Food Labeling Chaos: The Case for Reform," *Center for Science in the Public Interest* (March 2010): http://cspinet.org/new/pdf/food_labeling_chaos_report.pdf (accessed September 28, 2011).

Sinatra, Stephen. "Dr. Sinatra's Story: From Witnessing My Mom's Dangerous, Diabetic Blood Sugar Swings to Unmasking the Cholesterol and Low-Fat Myths," in *Sugar Shock! How Sweets and Simple Carbs Can Derail Your Life—And How You Can Get Back on Track,* 17–27. New York: Berkley Publishing Group, 2007.

————. Phone conversations about the sugar-heart disease connection with Connie Bennett, and follow-up e-mails to confirm quotes.

Skerrett, P.J. "Is Fructose Bad For You?" *Harvard Health Blog* (April 26, 2011): http://www.health.harvard .edu/blog/is-fructose-bad-for-you-201104262425 (accessed September 28, 2011).

Skinner, Ginger. "High-Fructose Corn Syrup is Not 'Corn Sugar,'" *Consumer Reports* (March 9, 2011): http://news.consumerreports.org/health/2011/03/high-fructose-corn-syrup-is-not-corn-sugar-corn -refiners-association-.html (accessed September 28, 2011).

Slattery, Martha L. et al. "Energy Balance, Insulin-Related Genes and Risk of Colon and Rectal Cancer," *International Journal of Cancer* 115, no. 1 (May 2005): 148–154. http://onlinelibrary.wiley.com /doi/10.1002/ijc.20843/full (accessed October 16, 2011).

Smith, Jeffrey. "The Health Dangers of Genetically Modified Foods," Video. http://www.youtube.com /watch?v=94d-KVorSHM (accessed September 30, 2011).

Smith, Mark and Brad LaTour. "How to Burst for Wellness," *Sweeter Holiday Summit with Connie Bennett* Session #14. Paid teleseminar program (Nov. 30, 2010): http://InstantTeleseminar .com/?eventid=16230153 (accessed September 30, 2011).

Sohn, Emily. "Plastic Water Bottles May Pose Health Hazard," *Discovery Channel* (April 28, 2009): http:// dsc.discovery.com/news/2009/04/28/water-bottles-health.html (accessed September 28, 2011).

Somer, Elizabeth. *Food & Mood: The Complete Guide to Eating Well and Feeling Your Best.* New York: Holt Paperbacks, 1999.

Somov, Pavel. "Craving Control for Overeating: Strategies and Tactics," *Huffington Post* (April 1, 2009): http://www.huffingtonpost.com/pavel-somov/craving-control-for-overe_b_181576.html (accessed September 28, 2011).

Stattin, P. et al. "Prospective Study of Hyperglycemia and Cancer Risk," *Diabetes Care* 30, no. 3 (March 2007): 561–567. http://www.ncbi.nlm.nih.gov/pubmed/17327321 (abstract accessed October 1, 2011).

Stinnett, Kyla. "Benefits of Meditation," *The Chopra Center*: http://www.chopra.com/agni/aug10 /benefits (accessed September 28, 2011).

St. Onge, Marie-Pierre et al. "Short Sleep Duration Increases Energy Intakes but Does Not Change Energy Expenditure in Normal-Weight Individuals," *American Journal of Clinical Nutrition* 94, no. 2 (June 29, 2011): 410–416. http://www.ajcn.org/content/94/2/410 (abstract accessed October 16, 2011).

Stöppler, Melissa Conrad. "Menstrual Cramps (Dysmenorrhea)," *MedicineNet.com:* http://www .medicinenet.com/menstrual_cramps/article.htm (accessed September 28, 2011).

Straus, Stephen E. "Statement before the Senate Appropriations Subcommittee on Labor, DHHS, Education, and Related Agencies," *National Center for Complementary and Alternative Medicine* (March 28, 2000): http://nccam.nih.gov/about/offices/od/directortestimony/032800.htm (accessed September 28, 2011).

Strickland, Dawn. E-mail correspondence for "Dawn Strickland's Sweet Success Story: How Coaching with Connie Helped Me Finally Quit Sugar for Good."

Tabata, Izumi et al. "Effects of Moderate-Intensity Endurance and High-Intensity Intermittent Training on Anaerobic Capacity and 'VO$_{2max}$,'" *Medicine & Science in Sports & Exercise* 28, no. 10 (October 1996): 1327–1330. http://journals.lww.com/acsm-msse/Abstract/1996/10000/Effects_of_moderate_intensity _endurance_and.18.aspx (abstract accessed September 30, 2011).

———. "Metabolic Profile of High Intensity Intermittent Exercises," *Medicine & Science in Sports & Exercise* 29, no. 3 (March 1997): 390–395. http://journals.lww.com/acsm-msse/Abstract/1997/03000 /Metabolic_profile_of_high_intensity_intermittent.15.aspx (abstract accessed September 28, 2011).

Tapping Solution (Try It on Everything): http://www.thetappingsolution.com/ (accessed October 16, 2011).

Taubes, Gary. "Is Sugar Toxic?" *The New York Times* (April 13, 2011): http://www.nytimes .com/2011/04/17/magazine/mag-17Sugar-t.html (accessed September 28, 2011).

———. "What If It's All Been a Big Fat Lie?" *The New York Times* (July 7, 2002): http://www.nytimes.com/2002/07/07/magazine/what-if-it-s-all-been-a-big-fat-lie.html (accessed September 28, 2011).

Taylor, Glenda. "The New Atkins Diet," *Livestrong* (October 12, 2010): http://www.livestrong.com/article/277529-the-new-atkins-diet/ (accessed September 28, 2011).

Teitelbaum, Jacob. *Beat Sugar Addiction Now!: The Cutting-Edge Program That Cures Your Type of Sugar Addiction and Puts You on the Road to Feeling Great—and Losing Weight!* United States: Fair Winds Press, 2010.

Thomley, Barbara et al. "Effects of a Brief, Comprehensive, Yoga-Based Program on Quality of Life and Biometric Measures in an Employee Population: A Pilot Study," *Explore* 7, no. 1 (January/February 2011): 27–29. http://www.explorejournal.com/article/S1550-8307%2810%2900219-3/fulltext (accessed September 28, 2011).

Thompson, Andrea. "Misleading Food Labels to Get Makeover: FDA Developing Restrictions For Front-of-Package Claims," MSNBC.com (March 15, 2010): http://www.msnbc.msn.com/id/35839186/ns/health-diet_and_nutrition/t/misleading-food-labels-get-makeover (accessed September 28, 2011).

Toman, Barbara. "Celiac Disease: On the Rise," *Discovery's Edge: Mayo Clinic's Online Research Magazine* (January 9, 2010): http://discoverysedge.mayo.edu/celiac-disease/ (accessed November 23, 2011).

Trugman, Avraham Arieh. "Jewish Meditation," Video. (December 2, 2008): http://www.youtube.com/watch?v=WORwKc_IAQc (accessed September 28, 2011).

U.S. Food and Drug Administration. "Acrylamide Questions and Answers": http://www.fda.gov/food/foodsafety/foodcontaminantsadulteration/chemicalcontaminants/acrylamide/ucm053569.htm (accessed September 30, 2011).

Van De Grift, Deborah et al. "Life Coaching: Pursue Your Passions, Move Your Life to a Better Direction," *Gab with the Gurus with Connie Bennett* (June 10, 2008): http://www.blogtalkradio.com/stopsugarshock/2008/06/10/life-coaching-pursue-your-passions-move-your-life-to-a-better-direction-panel-of-experts (accessed September 30, 2011).

Van der Heijden, A.A. et al. "A Prospective Study of Breakfast Consumption and Weight Gain Among U.S. Men," *Obesity (Silver Spring)* 15 (February 2007): 2463–2469. http://www.nature.com/oby/journal/v15/n10/full/oby2007292a.html (abstract accessed October 16, 2011).

Velez-Mitchell, Jane. "Jane Velez-Mitchell: Our 'Addict Nation,'" *Gab with the Gurus with Connie Bennett* (February 18, 2011): http://www.blogtalkradio.com/gabwiththegurus/2011/02/18/jane-velez-mitchell-our-addict-nation (accessed October 7, 2011).

———. Follow-up e-mails with publicist to confirm quotes for sidebar, "Sweet Success Story: Living Without Alcohol or Sugar in an 'Addict Nation.'"

Vidinsky, Kate. "UCSF Lecture on Sugar & Obesity Goes Viral as Experts Confront Health Crisis," *UCSF News Center* (March 11, 2010): http://www.ucsf.edu/news/2010/03/3222/ucsf-lecture-sugar-and-obesity-goes-viral-experts-confront-health-cri (accessed September 30, 2011).

Vienne, Veronique. *The Art of Doing Nothing: Simple Ways to Make Time for Yourself.* New York: Clarkson Potter Publishers, 1998.

Virgin, JJ. "Five Fun After-School Snacks," *Mom Logic* (August 29, 2010): http://www.momlogic .com/2010/08/five_fun_after-school_snacks.php (accessed September 30, 2011).

———. "Middle Aged and Gaining Weight? Doesn't Have to Be That Way!" Video. (December 1, 2009): http://www.youtube.com/watch?v=xxfykYxlA5E (accessed September 30, 2011).

———. "Secrets to Be Fit, Toned, Slim, Sexy & Sleeveless With Celebrity Wellness Expert," *Gab with the Gurus with Connie Bennett* (May 12, 2010): http://www.blogtalkradio.com/gabwiththe gurus/2010/05/12/secrets-to-be-fit-toned-slim-sexy-sleeveless-with- (accessed September 30, 2011).

Vitale, Joe. "Healing with Ho'oponopono," *Dr. Joe Vitale's Law of Attraction Blog* (August 5, 2010): http:// blog.mrfire.com/healing-with-hooponopono/ (accessed September 30, 2011).

———. "Joe Vitale on the Law of Attraction, Forgiveness & More," *Gab with the Gurus with Connie Bennett* (January 7, 2011): http://www.blogtalkradio.com/gabwiththegurus/2011/01/07/joe-vitale-on-the -law-of-attraction-forgiveness-mo (accessed September 30, 2011).

Vitale, Joe, and Ihaleakala Hew Len. *Zero Limits: The Secret Hawaiian System for Wealth, Health, Peace, and More.* Hoboken, New Jersey: John Wiley & Sons, 2008.

Vos, Miriam. "Caloric Sweetener Consumption and Dyslipidemia Among U.S. Adults," *Journal of the American Medical Association* 303, no. 15 (April 21, 2010): 1490–1497. http://www.ncbi.nlm.nih.gov /pmc/articles/PMC3045262/pdf/nihms216565.pdf (accessed October 14, 2011).

———. "High Sugar consumption May Increase Risk Factors for Heart Disease in American Teenagers," *Science Daily* (January 11, 2011): http://www.sciencedaily.com/releases/2011/01/110110164929.htm (accessed November 23, 2011.)

———. "Medical Horizon [Analysis of Medical Discoveries by Emory Doctors]: Added Sugars Increase Heart Disease Risk Factors," Video. (April 20, 2010): http://www.youtube.com/watch?v=MPTTsltWfX8 (accessed October 1, 2011).

Walker, Cheryl. "Psychologist Finds Self-Compassion Helps People Cope with Failure," *Wake Forest University* (August 22, 2005): http://www.wfu.edu/wfunews/2005/082205l.html (accessed September 30, 2011).

Wansink, Brian. *Mindless Eating: Why We Eat More Than We Think.* New York: Bantam Books, 2010.

———. Mindless Eating website: http://mindlesseating.org/faq.php (accessed October 16, 2011).

Wansink, Brian and Jeffrey Sobal. "Mindless Eating: The 200 Daily Food Decisions We Overlook," *Environment and Behavior* 39, no. 1 (January 2007): 106–123. http://eab.sagepub.com/content/39/1/106 .abstract (abstract accessed October 16, 2011).

Wansink, Brian et al. "Exploring Comfort Food Preferences Across Age and Gender," *Physiology & Behavior* 79 (2003): 739–747. http://mindlesseating.org/pdf/downloads/ComfortFood-P&B_2003.pdf (accessed October 1, 2011).

Waterhouse, J. et al. "Effects of Music Tempo upon Submaximal Cycling Performance," *Scandinavian Journal of Medicine & Science in Sports* 20, no. 4 (August 20, 2010): 662–669. http://www.ncbi.nlm.nih .gov/pubmed/19793214 (accessed September 30, 2011).

Watts, Merritt. "Healthy Bites: Eat Like…Jillian Michaels," *Self* (August 5, 2009) http://www.self.com/fooddiet/blogs/healthybites/2009/08/eat-like-jillian-michaels.html (accessed August 6, 2011).

Weatherby, Craig. "Omega-3 Lack May Fuel Sugar Cravings: Marine Omega-3s Called a More Effective Remedy than Plant Counterparts," *Vital Choices Newsletter* 2, no. 28 (June 10, 2005): http://newsletter.vitalchoice.com/e_article000411963.cfm?x=b53jlSr,b1WDbhNQ,w (accessed September 30, 2011).

Wedro, Benjamin. "Dehydration," *MedicineNet.com:* http://www.medicinenet.com/dehydration/article.htm#tocb (accessed September 30, 2011).

Weil, Andrew. "Q & A Library: Is Coconut Oil Good for You," *DrWeil.com* (March 21, 2005): http://www.drweil.com/drw/u/id/QAA316479 (accessed September 30, 2011).

———. "Turmeric Health Benefits: Have a Happy New Year with Turmeric," *Huffington Post* (December 28, 2010): http://www.huffingtonpost.com/andrew-weil-md/turmeric-health-have-a-happy-new-year_b_798328.html (accessed September 30, 2011).

———. "What Is Chia?" *DrWeil.com* (May 15, 2006): http://www.drweil.com/drw/u/QAA365093/Chia-for-Health.html (accessed September 28, 2011).

Weise, Elizabeth. "Is Organic Always the Best Pick When It Comes to Buying Food?" *USA Today* (December 22, 2010): http://www.usatoday.com/yourlife/food/2010-12-21-Organics21_CV_N.htm (accessed September 30, 2011).

Weiss, Edward et al. "Weight Regain in U.S. Adults Who Experienced Substantial Weight Loss, 1999–2002," *American Journal of Preventive Medicine* 33, no. 1 (July 2007): 34–40. http://www.ajpm-online.net/article/S0749-3797%2807%2900163-8/abstract (accessed September 30, 2011).

Westman, Eric C. et al. *New Atkins for a New You: The Ultimate Diet for Shedding Weight and Feeling Great.* New York: Touchstone; Original edition (March 2, 2010).

Williamson, Marianne. *A Course in Weight Loss: 21 Spiritual Lessons for Surrendering Your Weight Forever.* Carlsbad, CA: Hay House, 2010.

———. *Illuminata: A Return to Prayer.* New York: Riverhead Trade, 1995.

———. "Marianne Williamson: Surrender Your Weight Using Spiritual Lessons," *Gab with the Gurus with Connie Bennett* (January 6, 2011): http://www.blogtalkradio.com/gabwiththegurus/2011/01/06/marianne-williamson-surrender-your-weight-using-sp (accessed October 7, 2011).

Wolfe, David. "Superfoods Guru David 'Avocado' Wolfe on Cacao & More," *Gab with the Gurus with Connie Bennett.* Replay of interview on March 3, 2009: http://www.blogtalkradio.com/gabwiththegurus/2011/10/17/superfoods-guru-david-avocado-wolfe-on-cacao-more (accessed October 17, 2011).

Wolpert, Stuart. "Dieting Doesn't Work," *UCLA Magazine* (April 4, 2007): http://magazine.ucla.edu/exclusives/dieting_no-go/ (accessed September 30, 2011).

Woo, Elaine. "Gordon Shaw, 72; Linked Music to Thinking," *Los Angeles Times* (May 1, 2005): http://articles.latimes.com/2005/may/01/local/me-shaw1 (accessed September 30, 2011).

Woolverton, Frederick. "Beat Your Addictions with Dr. Frederick Woolverton," *Gab with the Gurus with Connie Bennett:* http://www.blogtalkradio.com/gabwiththegurus/2010/08/17/beat-your-addictions-with-dr-frederick-woolverton-1 (accessed October 7, 2011).

World Health Organization. "Frequently Asked Questions—Acrylamide in food": http://www.who.int /foodsafety/publications/chem/acrylamide_faqs/en/ (accessed September 30, 2011).

World's Healthiest Foods, The. "What Is the Glycemic Index?": http://www.whfoods.com/genpage .php?tname=faq&dbid=32 (accessed September 28, 2011).

Yang, Qing. "Gain Weight by 'Going Diet?' Artificial Sweeteners and the Neurobiology of Sugar Cravings," *Yale Journal of Biology and Medicine* 83, no. 2 (June 2010): 101–108. http://www.ncbi.nlm.nih .gov/pmc/articles/PMC2892765/ (accessed October 16, 2011).

Yang, Sarah. "Nearly One-Third of the Calories in the US Diet Come from Junk Food, Researcher Finds," *Berekely.edu* (June 1, 2004): http://berkeley.edu/news/media/releases/2004/06/01_usdiet.shtml (accessed November 23, 2011).

Yoga Journal Press Release. "Yoga Journal Releases 2008 'Yoga in America' Market Study: Practitioner Spending Grows to Nearly $6 Billion a Year," *Yoga Journal* (February 26, 2008): http://www.yogajournal .com/media/originals/YJ_PR_YogaAmerica.pdf (accessed September 30, 2011).

Young, Simon. "How to Increase Serotonin in the Human Brain Without Drugs," *Journal of Psychiatry & Neuroscience* 32, no. 6 (November 2007): 394–399. http://www.ncbi.nlm.nih.gov/pmc/articles /PMC2077351/ (accessed Oct. 13, 2011).

Yuhara H. et al. "Is Diabetes Mellitus an Independent Risk Factor for Colon Cancer and Rectal Cancer?" *The American Journal of Gastroenterology* 106, no. 11 (November 2011): 1911–1921. http://www.ncbi .nlm.nih.gov/pubmed?term=Hiroki%20Yuhara%20and%20colon (abstract accessed November 21, 2011).

Zajac, Andrew. "FDA Issues Warning on Food Labels: Seventeen Companies are Asked to Change Misleading Claims on Health and Nutrition," *Los Angeles Times* (March 4, 2010): http://articles.latimes .com/2010/mar/04/business/la-fi-fda-food-labels4-2010mar04 (accessed September 30, 2011).

Zelman, Kathleen M. "The Glycemic Index Diet (Low Glycemic Diet)," *WebMD*: http://www.webmd .com/diet/features/glycemic-index-diet (accessed September 28, 2011).

Zeratsky, Katherine. "Monosodium Glutamate (MSG): Is It Harmful?" *MayoClinic.com* (January 9, 2010): http://www.mayoclinic.com/health/monosodium-glutamate/AN01251 (accessed October 15, 2011).

Zimmerman, Eilene. "Winning the Nutrition Game, With Help from a Coach," *The New York Times* (April 22, 2007): http://www.nytimes.com/2007/04/22/business/yourmoney/22food.html? _r=4&scp=1&sq=nutrition%20coach&st=cse (accessed September 30, 2011).

Zimmerman, Stephanie. Phone calls and e-mail follow-ups for "Stephanie Zimmerman's Sweet Success Story: How I Lost & Kept Off 220 Pounds."

# INDEX

# Index

## B

Balsamic Dressings, *213*
Beans and legumes, 193–194
*Beat Sugar Addiction Now!* (Teitelbaum), 73, 235
Beverages
    alcoholic. *See* Alcohol
    caffeine in, 99, 111
    shopping list, 206
    sweetening during phase-out period, 99–100
Beyond Sugar Shock Freedom SparkTeam. *See*
    SparkPeople (and SparkTeam)
Big Preventable Killers, 21–34. *See also* Cancer;
    Diabetes
    about: overview of, 21–22
    heart disease, 24–26
    sugar/quickie carbs impacting body, 22–24.
        *See also* Health
Bison Burger, *227*
Bittman, Mark, 36
Biziou, Barbara, 125
Block Center for Integrative Cancer Treatment, 28
Block, Gladys, Ph.D., xviii
Block, Keith I., M.D., 28
Blogging, 165, 166
Blood sugar. *See also* Diabetes; Insulin
    cancer and, 27–28
    carb snacks and, 111, 139
    coconut oil and, 147
    coffee and, 158
    curbing strategy, 99
    discovering causes of issues with, 73
    excessive, sugar/carbs and, xxii, 8, 23
    imbalance, 22–23
    importance of breakfast for, 104
    low, xxviii, 6, 7, 23
    metabolic syndrome and, 30, 33–34
    obesity and, 30
    omega-3s and, 144
    spiking, 8
    stabilizing, to avoid cravings, 97, 99, 141–142,
        144, 147, 158
Body
    choosing smarter habits/better food behavior.
        *See* Week Two
    eating wholesome food for. *See* Eating, new
        way of; Recipes; Week Four
    Mirror Love Affirmations, 83–84
    starting love affair with, 82–85
    writing love letter to, 84–85
Bondage. *See* Addiction to sugar; Five Stages of
    Sugar Bondage

Book overview, xv–xxv
    backstory, xxii–xxiii
    S.A.D. world and, xviii–xix
    symptoms of "Right Readers," xvii–xviii
    terms defined, xx–xxii, 8
    what to expect, xix–xx
Books, 235–236
Bowden, Jonny, Ph.D., C.N.S, 142, 158
Breakfast
    importance of, 104
    recipes for, *219, 226*
    S.A.D. to SWEET choices, 104
Break Free of Your Sugar Addiction in 6 Weeks
    Program, 9–10, 243
Buddhist Metta Meditation, 179–180
Bursting, 113–114

## C

Caffeine, 99, 111
Calories
    low-fat or low-calorie foods and, 37, 101–102
    from sweeteners, 25
Cancer
    beef, CLA and, 239
    coconut oil and, 146–147
    feeding on sugar, 27
    omega-3s and, 144, 145
    phytochemicals and, 136
    sugar impacting, 27–28
Carbs (much-like-sugar, toxic, quickie)
    affirmation for eliminating, 147
    benefits of eliminating, xix–xx
    comfort foods and, 38–39
    comfort pseudo-foods, 38–39
    danger of, 8
    eliminating, 147–151
    gluten sensitivity and, 148
    low-fat or low-calorie foods and, 37, 101–102
    making you fat and sick, 22–24
    as "metabolic bullies," 33–34
    *natural* foods and, xix–xx, 37
    negative effects summary, xx–xxi
    other risky white foods, 31
    processed foods and weight gain, 28–29
    S.A.D. and, xxi–xxii
    S.A.D. Bondage and, 41–42
    spiking sugar levels, 8
    sugar-fat mix and, 36–37
    throwing body into crisis, 22–24
    whole grains in place of, 147–149, 202–203

# Index

# NOTES

# NOTES

# NOTES

# NOTES

# NOTES

# NOTES

# ACKNOWLEDGMENTS

*"Feeling gratitude and not expressing it is
like wrapping a present and not giving it."*

— WILLIAM ARTHUR WARD

Now that *Beyond Sugar Shock* is finally coming to life 14 years after I grudgingly quit sugar on doctor's orders, I'm honored, humbled, and awed when I think about the enormous amount of generosity, support, and encouragement that I've received over the years from thousands of brave, committed, dedicated individuals around the world.

Indeed, as with my first book, *Sugar Shock!*, I discovered that if you seek to create an engaging, healing, uplifting, life-changing book, you have to rely on the blessings, research, and contributions of thousands of people. So my gratitude list is long.

First and foremost, I bow my head and curtsy in gratitude galore to thousands of sugar and carb addicts whom I've had the pleasure of helping either on- or offline (via phone or in person) since late 2002.

In particular, I give big, appreciative cyber hugs to my many successful coaching clients, readers of *Sugar Shock!*, and the members of my various online communities, especially the original KickSugar support group on Yahoo and early "guinea pigs" of this book's program (Jennifer, Ju, Lisa B., Lee Anne, Linda, Lisa, Lynn, and Suzanne).

Furthermore, I'm beholden to thousands of sugaraholics, who joined my Break Free of Your Sugar Addiction in 6 Weeks Program from its modest beginnings in 2002 to my current signature Sugar Freedom Now Course, this book's companion program.

I'm honored that you, my target audience, honestly shared your worries, frustrations, and concerns, as well as what you needed to release your sugar habit for good. And thanks to Myra Pinkham and Keri Gans, R.D., for being instrumental in KickSugar's early years.

Meanwhile, more gratitude goes to volunteer coordinators and fans of the Beyond Sugar Shock Freedom SparkTeam on SparkPeople, Smart Habits Fans on Facebook, and the Beyond Sugar Shock community on TheBlogFrog.

As an author and journalist, I'm also deeply grateful to the many warm, dedicated, kind, professional people at my publisher, Hay House, especially the charming, forward-thinking editor Patricia Gift, whose enthusiasm about publishing a six-week, Mind-Body-Spirit, kick-sugar plan made this book a reality.

It's been a joy and a wonderful growing experience to work with Patty and the sweet, thoughtful Sally Mason, whose insightful, probing questions forced me to provide you with even juicier, quality content to help you break free.

I'm also especially thankful and indebted to the inspiring Cheryl Richardson, whose fabulous book, *Take Time for Your Life*—required reading for my life-coaching training at the Institute for Professional Excellence in Coaching—lured me to attend a profound, life-changing Hay House Movers & Shakers program.

At that event, I had the awesome opportunity and transformational experience of meeting my long-time heroine, the amazing Louise L. Hay, whose *You Can Heal Your Life* first inspired me years ago; and Hay House's remarkable visionary leader Reid Tracy, whose encouraging remarks and big thoughts always spur me on.

I'm also filled with tremendous admiration and heartfelt appreciation to the talented, dedicated, freelance editor Stephanie Abarbanel, who showed up out of the blue just when I needed her. Stephanie, thank you so much for your consistently brilliant direction, invaluable guidance, and vital editing suggestions to make this program flow better so I could truly help readers of this book easily break free of their sugar addiction.

Furthermore, I'm thrilled to have a sharp, amiable, encouraging literary agent and energetic champion in Wendy Sherman. You're amazing, Wendy, and I'm blessed to have you cheering me on and representing me so I can reach and help millions around the world.

This book also owes its life to the astute veteran journalist and broadcaster Dana Kennedy, founder of the www.AYearWithoutCandy.com blog. Dana, thanks so much for emphatically insisting that the time was right for my second book.

I'm also honored that nutritionist/exercise physiologist Jill Lane, C.N.C., took time to provide the Meal Plan and recipes and answer my many health questions.

I'm also very thankful to Joshua Rosenthal, founder and director of the Institute for Integrative Nutrition for contributing the amazing foreword to this book and to Annie Wong, Julia Argenti, and Robert Notter, also of IIN.

# Acknowledgments

In addition, I'm grateful to Bruce Schneider, Luke Iorio, Deborah Van De Grift, Fredi Baker, and Kimberly Bagwell of iPEC, for the amazing coach training you provided.

I'm also in awe of the generous, always-encouraging, knowledgeable sugar experts Nancy Appleton, Ph.D.; Ann Louise Gittleman, Ph.D., C.N.S.; and Jacob Teitelbaum, M.D., who supported me and offered vital guidance while I developed expertise as a Sugar Freedom Coach—even though they have sugar books of their own. What generosity!

I'm also thrilled to have had the pivotal encouragement of the brilliant, big-hearted, generous JJ Virgin, Ph.D. and Diana Kirschner, Ph.D.; as well as John Assaraf, Russ Bianchi, Joe Vitale, David Rourke, Ph.D., Carol Look, Lauren Frances, and Debra Berndt. Not only did you appear on my *Gab with the Gurus Radio Show,* but you all gave me so much in so many other ways. I cannot thank you enough!

Many thanks also go to the amazing supporters Arielle Ford; Mark Patrick; Joyce Schwarz; Brian Alman, Ph.D.; Jean Kristeller, Ph.D.; Ken Druck, Ph.D.; Lilian Cheung, D.Sc., R.D.; Jeffrey Morrison, M.D., C.N.S.; and Bernie Siegel, M.D., who all graciously shared transformational ideas on my *Gab with the Gurus Radio Show* or other programs so I could inspire you.

And more gratitude goes to gurus Steve G. Jones, Natalie Ledwell, Nicolas Ortner, Jane Velez-Mitchell, Marci Shimoff, Janet Atwood, Hale Dwoskin, Paul Hoffman, Marina Kamen, Rafael Cushnir, and David Harp.

I'm also grateful to transformational Hay House authors and speakers Marianne Williamson, Doreen Virtue, Chris Downie, Deborah King, Colette Baron-Reid, Lauren Mackler, Caroline Sutherland, and Peter Rodger, Darren Weissman, D.C., and Michael A. Snyder, M.D., who all graciously took time out to appear on my *Gab with the Gurus Radio Show.*

Furthermore, I'm indebted to the many other fabulous Hay House people, including Carina Sammartino, Laura Koch, Nancy Levin, John Thompson, Richelle Zizian, Lindsay McGinty, Tiffani Alberto, Gail Gonzalez, Diane Ray, Karen Stone, Shelley Anderson, Wioleta Gramek, Heather Tate, Donna Abate, Darcy Duval, Tricia Breidenthal, Johanne Mahaffey, and Christy Salinas.

Many thanks also go Gale Maleskey, M.S., R.D., for helping to decipher medical studies and information. I'm also thankful to health researchers/writers Carey Rossi, Sandra Gordon, Mark Fuerst, Rachel Martin, and Beverly Burmeier.

I'm also grateful to my interns/research assistants Sara Best, Shanté Fenique King, Cally J. Schulte, Scott Henneboehle, Carrie Thompson, Ann Cook, and Hollis Templeton, as well as Hilary Powell, Chris Gray, Jeremy Gordon, and Lana Birbrair.

On a personal health front, I'm deeply grateful to the brilliant nutritionist Dr. Gittleman for helping me discover, while on deadline for this book, that I was being *Zapped* (also the name of her great book) by electromagnetic radiation (EMF) due to the very long hours I spent in front of my computer writing and rewriting this manuscript or interviewing experts on my cordless phone. Thanks to you, Ann Louise, as well as Matthew Maletzke, Jo-Anne Piazza, Shauna Robitaille, Marilee Tolen, Kaitlyn Keyt, and Kerry Crofton, Ph.D., for helping me rapidly reclaim my health so I could finish this book.

I'd also like to thank early supporters of *Sugar Shock!*, including Mehmet Oz, M.D., who said kind words about it; Stephen T. Sinatra, M.D., who served as contributing author; and Nicholas Perricone, M.D., who wrote the foreword to it.

I'm also honored that Fred Pescatore, M.D.; Jonny Bowden, Ph.D., C.N.S.; Christiane Northrup, M.D.; Kathy Smith; Oz Garcia, Ph.D.; and blogger Jimmy Moore were among the many who endorsed the book.

More acknowledgments go to members of the media, who first helped spread the word about *Sugar Shock!*, especially *TIME* magazine's Andrea Sachs and Amy Oscar of *Woman's World.*

In addition, I'm grateful to the inspirational speakers, life-changing authors, marketers/mentors Lisa Sasevich, Lisa Cherney, Andrea J. Lee, Steve and Bill Harrison, Peggy McColl, Ali Brown, Barbara DeAngelis, Lorrie Morgan-Ferrero, Michele Pariza Wacek (Michele PW), Mike Koenigs, Janet Goldstein, Elizabeth Marshall, Christine Kloser, Lynne Klippel, Alex Mandossian, Jack Canfield, Mark Victor Hansen, Rick Frishman, Robert G. Allen, Brian Jud, Matthew Bennett, Randy Gilbert, Cindy Ratzlaff, Gregory Godek, T. Harv Eker, Seth Godin, Mari Smith, Chris Brogan, Joel Comm, Dan Janal, Michael Stelzner, Denise Wakeman, Shama Kabani, Andy Wibbels, Mitch Meyerson, Timothy Ferriss, Michael Port, Geneen Roth, Gary Vaynerchuk, Deepak Chopra, Elizabeth Gilbert, Katharine Woodward Thomas, Claire Zammit, Alison Armstrong, and Garland Landrith, Ph.D.

I also appreciate the artistic Carla Alvarez for her work on my Beyond Sugar Shock and Sweeter Holiday Summit websites, and Rose Petruzzi, who created the playful "Sugar Shrew" Connie cartoon character years ago.

What's more, I'm grateful to Jill Baron, M.D.; Lohkmin Lee; Deborah Voorhees; and Nancy Hancock, as well as my sister and brother-in-law.

Also, I'd like to pay tribute to the late pioneers Jack LaLanne, William Dufty, and Robert C. Atkins, M.D., for having the courage and dedication years ago to first warn people about the perils of sugar and simple carbs.

# Acknowledgments

And I applaud Gary Taubes, Jamie Oliver, Michael Pollan, Mark Bittman, Greg Critser, Morgan Spurlock, and Eric Schlosser; as well as Andrew Weil, M.D.; Joseph Mercola, D.O.; and Marion Nestle, Ph.D., M.P.H., for their important work educating people about good nutrition.

Thanks also to the Center for the Science in Public Interest, especially its co-founder and executive director Michael F. Jacobson, Ph.D., and valuable staff, Jeff Cronin and Margo Wootan. Your organization does such valuable advocacy work on behalf of all Americans.

This *Beyond Sugar Shock* Gratitude List wouldn't be complete without a huge nod of appreciation to Whole Foods Market, Vital Choice, Westerly Natural Market, and farmers with scrumptious organic vegetables and grass-fed meat, etc., for keeping me well nourished. Yummy!

And what would I have done without my cherished Equinox Fitness membership, as well as my X-iser and Malibu Pilates machines, which all kept me naturally high?

God or Universal Intelligence, I also humbly thank you for continually leading, guiding, and directing me to write this book so I could serve people around the world.

And you, dear readers, of course, I'm very grateful to all of you, for being here. I treasure you and believe in you.

Sugar and carb addicts of all sizes and shapes, thank you so much for putting your trust and confidence in me.

And make sure to connect on Facebook, my blog, website, and our SparkTeam so I can hear your Sweet Success Stories or answer your questions.

# ABOUT THE AUTHOR

Connie Bennett, C.H.H.C., C.P.C., A.C.C., is an acclaimed, engaging, transformational speaker, certified health coach, certified life coach, journalist, and charismatic former sugar addict, who playfully pokes fun at her past as a "Sugar Shrew."

She is the author of the best-selling book *Sugar Shock! How Sweets and Simple Carbs Can Derail Your Life—And How You Can Get Back on Track*, with Stephen T. Sinatra, M.D. The book has been praised by Mehmet Oz, M.D.; Christiane Northrup, M.D.; Marilu Henner; Joseph Mercola, D.O., and many others.

Connie is dedicated to helping people worldwide to easily, effortlessly release their sugar addiction and other bad habits. She hosts the *Gab with the Gurus Radio Show*, for which she interviews celebrities and best-selling authors in a variety of fields.

She attended the Institute for Integrative Nutrition (IIN), the Institute for Professional Excellence in Coaching (iPEC), and the Vision Board Institute. She also took classes at the Natural Gourmet Institute for Health & Culinary Arts and at other culinary schools.

Connie's sad-to-sweet journey reached a low point in 1998, when she was plagued by 44 ailments, including mood swings, fatigue, brain fog, heart palpitations, and severe PMS. After quitting sugar and quickie carbs on doctor's orders, all her ailments vanished, and she regained her health and sense of humor. In 2002, Connie founded her first kick-sugar program, which evolved into this book and her signature Sugar Freedom Now Course, this book's companion program.

Connie is passionate about—and often "fills up" on—bicycling, Zumba Fitness, intenSati, bursting, tennis, Ping-Pong, skiing, long walks, her X-iser, gratitude, Tapping, meditation, Ho'oponopono, eating organically, and positive people.

Connect with Connie on her website at www.BeyondSugarShock.com, her blog at www.SugarShockBlog.com, her radio show at www.GabWithTheGurus.com, and her Sugar Freedom Now Course at www.BreakFreeWithConnie.com.

# HAY HOUSE TITLES OF RELATED INTEREST

*YOU CAN HEAL YOUR LIFE, the movie,* starring Louise L. Hay & Friends
(available as a 1-DVD program and an expanded 2-DVD set)
Watch the trailer at: **www.LouiseHayMovie.com**

*THE SHIFT, the movie,*
starring Dr. Wayne W. Dyer
(available as a 1-DVD program and an expanded 2-DVD set)
Watch the trailer at: **www.DyerMovie.com**

• • •

*THE BELLY FAT CURE: Discover the New Carb Swap System
and Lose 4 to 9 lbs. Every Week,* by Jorge Cruise

*CONSTANT CRAVING: What Your Food Cravings Mean
and How to Overcome Them,* by Doreen Virtue

*A COURSE IN WEIGHT LOSS: 21 Spiritual Lessons for
Surrendering Your Weight Forever,* by Marianne Williamson

*JUST AN OUNCE OF PREVENTION IS WORTH A POUND OF CURE: A Modern Guide
to Healthful Living from the Originator of the Blood-Type Diet,* by James D'Adamo

*THE SPARK: The 28-Day Breakthrough Plan for Losing Weight,
Getting Fit, and Transforming Your Life,* by Chris Downie

All of the above are available at your local bookstore,
or may be ordered by contacting Hay House (see next page).

• • •

We hope you enjoyed this Hay House book. If you'd like to receive our
online catalog featuring additional information on Hay House books and products,
or if you'd like to find out more about the Hay Foundation, please contact:

Hay House, Inc., P.O. Box 5100, Carlsbad, CA 92018-5100
(760) 431-7695 or (800) 654-5126
(760) 431-6948 (fax) or (800) 650-5115 (fax)
**www.hayhouse.com®** • **www.hayfoundation.org**

• • •

*Published and distributed in Australia by:* Hay House Australia Pty. Ltd., 18/36 Ralph St.,
Alexandria NSW 2015 • *Phone:* 612-9669-4299 • *Fax:* 612-9669-4144 • www.hayhouse.com.au

*Published and distributed in the United Kingdom by:* Hay House UK, Ltd., 292B Kensal Rd.,
London W10 5BE • *Phone:* 44-20-8962-1230 • *Fax:* 44-20-8962-1239 • www.hayhouse.co.uk

*Published and distributed in the Republic of South Africa by:* Hay House SA (Pty), Ltd.,
P.O. Box 990, Witkoppen 2068 • *Phone/Fax:* 27-11-467-8904 • www.hayhouse.co.za

*Published in India by:* Hay House Publishers India, Muskaan Complex, Plot No. 3, B-2, Vasant Kunj,
New Delhi 110 070 • *Phone:* 91-11-4176-1620 • *Fax:* 91-11-4176-1630 • www.hayhouse.co.in

*Distributed in Canada by:* Raincoast, 9050 Shaughnessy St., Vancouver, B.C. V6P 6E5
*Phone:* (604) 323-7100 • *Fax:* (604) 323-2600 • www.raincoast.com

• • •

**Take Your Soul on a Vacation**

Visit **www.HealYourLife.com®** to regroup, recharge, and reconnect with your own magnificence.
Featuring blogs, mind-body-spirit news, and life-changing wisdom from Louise Hay and friends.

Visit **www.HealYourLife.com** today!

# Free Mind-Body-Spirit e-Newsletters

## From Hay House, the Ultimate Resource for Inspiration

**Be the first to know about Hay House's dollar deals, free downloads, special offers, affirmation cards, giveaways, contests, and more!**

 Get exclusive excerpts from our latest releases and videos from *Hay House Present Moments*.

 Enjoy uplifting personal stories, how-to articles, and healing advice, along with videos and empowering quotes, within *Heal Your Life*.

 Have an inspirational story to tell and a passion for writing? Sharpen your writing skills with insider tips from *Your Writing Life*.

Receive uplifting affirmations, empowering thoughts, and healing wisdom from *Louise Hay*.

Discover ways to overcome all obstacles with the inspiring words of *Dr. Wayne Dyer* to get your wishes fulfilled.

Get angelic, heavenly assistance for your everyday life from angel expert and lifelong clairvoyant *Doreen Virtue*.

Uncover the timeless secrets of life from *Gregg Braden* and discover the collective wisdom of our past.

**Get inspired, educate yourself, and share the wisdom!**
**Visit www.hayhouse.com to sign up today!**

 HAY HOUSE

 HAYHOUSE RADIO
*radio for your soul*

HealYourLife.com ♥

# Heal Your Life One Thought at a Time . . .
## on Louise's All-New Website!

*"Life is bringing me everything I need and more."*

— Louise Hay

**Come to HEALYOURLIFE.COM today** and meet the world's best-selling self-help authors; the most popular leading intuitive, health, and success experts; up-and-coming inspirational writers; and new like-minded friends who will share their insights, experiences, personal stories, and wisdom so you can heal your life and the world around you . . . one thought at a time.

## Here are just some of the things you'll get at HealYourLife.com:

- DAILY AFFIRMATIONS
- CAPTIVATING VIDEO CLIPS
- EXCLUSIVE BOOK REVIEWS
- AUTHOR BLOGS
- LIVE TWITTER AND FACEBOOK FEEDS
- BEHIND-THE-SCENES SCOOPS
- LIVE STREAMING RADIO
- "MY LIFE" COMMUNITY OF FRIENDS

**PLUS:**
FREE Monthly Contests and Polls
FREE BONUS gifts, discounts,
and newsletters

### Make It Your Home Page Today!
### www.HealYourLife.com®

## HEAL YOUR LIFE®